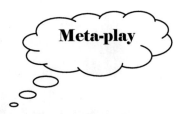

The Meta-play Method:™

Application of the Dynamic Behavior Theory of Autism (DBT-A)

Cooper R. Woodard, PhD, BCBA

ISBN 978-1-4675-2834-4

Contents

Preface and Acknowledgements   5

Part 1: Background, Basics, and a Primer on Meta-representation

Chapter 1: The Many Symptoms of Autism   12

Chapter 2: What We Know About Genes, Environment, Treatment, and Typical Early Development   24

Chapter 3: Explanations of the 9-month Revolution in Thinking: The Emergence of Imagination   40

Chapter 4: Imagination, Symbolism, and Pretend Play in Autism   58

Part 2: Emergence of the Dynamic Behavior Theory of Autism (DBT-A)

Chapter 5: Our Love-Hate Relationship with Psychoanalysis and Identification   75

Chapter 6: What It Means to Identify with an Object   90

Chapter 7: Movement Up the Continuum   106

Chapter 8: It Sounds Good, but is There Any Supporting Research?   123

Chapter 9: A Primer for Increasing the   143
Prevalence of Autism within a Population
and Future Directions

Part 3: Implementing the Meta-play Method

Chapter 10: The Meta-Play Method and
Other Models of Treatment   157

Chapter 11: Activities of the Meta-play
Method   162

Closing Comments   179

References   181

Preface and Acknowledgements

The path that has led to the writing of this book has been an unusual one, unlike the typical researcher in developmental disabilities. Almost 20 years ago, I accepted a position with a company that provides services to persons with developmental disabilities, mainly because my job conducting psychological evaluations for juveniles involved in the court system had been eliminated. Being a master's level psychologist, I needed supervision from someone with a doctoral degree, and as luck would have it, one of the finest researchers in the field, Dr. James Bodfish, was that person. For more than seven years, he taught me, guided me, listened to my questions, and supported my clinical, research, and often personal endeavors. I had no idea at the time how fortunate I was to have him as a mentor, and he is one of the people I would like to dedicate this book to, in that I owe him a debt of gratitude.

As budgets tightened in human services through the 1990's, I began to realize that I needed my own doctoral degree to be able to get the type of job I wanted. I returned to school and during my internship, good luck struck again as my mentor for clinical training was Dr. Mark Horner, a former student of Otto Kernberg. I was quickly introduced to the world of object relations theory, and shown how these key ideas were applied in a clinical setting. Once I understood the basics of this theory and saw how effective the tools were, I could not understand why the other interns in my program would not choose this orientation as their own. The object relations model was logical and not particularly difficult to understand, and the core idea that our relationships with our parents and significant others in our early world created a template for later relationships, seemed to make obvious sense to me. Dr. Mark Horner is the other person to whom I would like to dedicate this book, as he provided me with the foundational and clear understanding of these current psychoanalytic concepts.

I practiced for a year after receiving my doctoral degree, but found myself missing my work in developmental disabilities, as well as the northeast. I accepted a position as the clinical director for The Groden Center in Providence, Rhode Island, and I am quickly approaching my 10th anniversary. The Groden Center is part of a larger network of programs, created by Dr.'s June and Gerry Groden. These visionary clinicians started the program in the 1970's, employing a behavioral perspective but also remaining open to new and innovative ideas. The Groden Center school serves approximately 90 students ages 6-21, most of whom have an autism spectrum disorder (ASD) combined with significant behavioral and/or psychiatric issues. In my early years in my position as clinical director, I was looked at with curiosity by the other psychologists; "What is he doing here?" they undoubtedly thought. Most clinical directors who worked in this particular field have staunch behavioral backgrounds, and here I was with what most would consider the exact opposite, psychoanalytic training. Not only was my training in object relations theory often considered applicable to irrelevant "internal" behavior, most practitioners found it aversive due to a history of the psychoanalytic community incorrectly blaming the so-called "refrigerator" mother for the child's diagnosis of autism.

So I kept my background quiet, and instead earned the necessary credentials for the field by securing board certification as a behavior analyst (BCBA). It wasn't that I minded the behavioral approach; on the contrary, I have much respect for it and I have certainly made use of the tremendous amount of effective tools and interventions it offers. Behaviorism is currently the foundational perspective for some of the only interventions that have been found to actually lessen (and in certain situations ameliorate) symptoms associated with the early diagnosis of autism. These interventions need to be applied intensely during a child's formative years, but can change the course of the disorder in addition to lessening remaining problems if applied in later years. While this is both impressive and important, the behavioral approach limits its focus as the name implies; it is mainly and often solely concerned with what you and I can see ourselves and other *doing*. While thinking and feeling are not denied, these processes are not focused on by the behaviorist because they are private events not available for scientific verification. I would suggest that relying mainly on the behavioral orientation might inhibit a full understanding of how autism comes to be, and may be limiting our effectiveness.

So while behaviorism has made an immense contribution to the field, it has a sort of Achilles heel in that the tools necessary for understanding autism have become, to a great extent, needlessly "off limits." This situation leads us to the main purpose of this book: to demonstrate and explain how autism is an altered early trajectory of the development of an essential feature of mature, human thinking -- the ability to think "about" or imagine, in the broadest sense of the word. What I mean by this will hopefully become clearer as the reader progresses, but interestingly, this particular thinking ability is in itself, essential to understanding the main points contained in this volume. To be able to understand what autism is, the reader will need to imagine what it is like <u>not</u> to be able to imagine. This, I have found, is not an easy task for everyone who comes in contact with these ideas, mainly because this ability is such a core feature of who and what we are as thinking humans. We employ this ability with such ease and regularity, that imagining what it is like not to be able to imagine is difficult.

This book is an expansion of an article that I had published in 2011. While I was able to outline some of the main ideas in that article, space limitations did not allow for full explanations, and being a journal submission, I was not able to speculate on ideas to any great degree. Since those limits do not presently exist, we will begin with a discussion of what the diagnosis of autism actually entails, and more importantly, discuss the many symptoms not technically included in a diagnosis. These associated symptoms provide some essential clues to understanding autism, and will be returned to later in the book. Next, we will discuss the many fruitless attempts to identify the cause of autism, as well as the few basic facts we do currently have. This will lead us directly into a presentation of our core concepts and thesis, the development of early imaginative capacities which derive from the psychoanalytic process of part- to whole-object identification and internalization. Because this process is a multifaceted and complex one, we will need to consider the various sources of potential influence from both genetic and environmental sources. We will then discuss a range of research findings that support this theory, although since it is a new theory, the studies cited do so in a roundabout way. Finally, with these concepts understood, we can begin to speculate on why rates of this disorder appear to be increasing daily. I will not keep the reader in suspense; I will suggest that one source of influence increasing rates of autism comes from trends within our own culture, non-person engagement that is fueling a subtle change in who we are, how we think and behave, how we interact with and shape our own infants, and perhaps the thinking predispositions of our children.

So why do certain interventions seem to work and how can we use these ideas to maximize efforts? The last section of this book addresses these issues. If autism is in part, a culturally induced alteration of early development in the capacity to imagine, a non-completion of typical human-based identification and internalization, how can current, moderately effective interventions perhaps be made more effective? What types of research would provide further support for these ideas or disprove them? What does this theory mean to parents, and is it convincing enough to change behaviors and decisions about whether or not to have a child? I can only speculate on possible answers to these questions. However, I want to be clear when I note that there is no intent in these writings to blame the parent or throw the field of autism research into reverse. If someone shows that autism has a clear, single genetic or environmental cause, I will be more than pleased to retract the ideas contained in this book. But in the absence of such discoveries, it is my hope that by integrating multiple psychological perspectives, we will move closer to understanding autism and lessen the difficulties often associated with this diagnosis.

And finally, my sincerest thanks to my partner John Neill and my parents for listening to my endless discussions on this topic. And thanks to my sister Camaron Thomas, who spent many hours editing my notoriously poor grammar.

Cooper R. Woodard

Part 1: Background, Basics, and a Primer on Meta-representation

Chapter 1: The Many Symptoms of Autism

Autism is not an easy diagnosis to make, much less to understand from a conceptual standpoint. Unlike Attention Deficit Disorder (ADD) or the various presentations of depression, it is made up of a set of three subcategories that, despite our best efforts, do not seem to fit together in a comprehensive or meaningful way. Something like depression is relatively straight-forward; you are sad, not interested in things that used to be interesting, tired, and probably have trouble eating and/or sleeping. We can all identify with this grouping of symptoms, having most likely felt some form or another of depression at certain points in our lives. But autism is very different. It doesn't hit you late in life, it doesn't go away, there are no medications that effectively treat the core symptoms, and the subcategories don't really form one unique, coherent whole with which most people could identify. We don't have very good ideas about how it happens, where it comes from, or what can be done to prevent it, and because of this situation, most people keep it on the outskirts of their thinking, preferring to remain ignorant of the diagnosis until it touches their life. People typically don't know quite what it is when I tell them what I do for a living, but they seem to know it is bad and that autism is something that they don't want in their lives. I often get something like, "you must be a very special person to work with children like that." But my response is always the same; these are children and young adults without malice, shame, or most any of the less desirable traits that can accompany childhood and adolescence. They are, in fact, a pleasure and a joy with whom to spend time.

This book is an attempt to lessen at least some of the mystery that surrounds autism. Having worked with people with autism and other developmental disabilities for nearly 20 years, I have come to appreciate the varied faces of autism, as well as the courage, suffering, resilience, fear, strength and other traits and emotions that this diagnosis can elicit. As I mentioned in the preface, I was fortunate enough to have on-the-job behavioral training, as well as clinical training from a psychoanalytic orientation. While some might see these two perspectives as diametrically opposed to one another, I consider them complementary and the key to unraveling autism, which is one of the most complex and problematic psychological disorders of our time. To better understand autism, we will need to begin by defining it as best we can. This means not only looking at standard diagnostic criteria, but also any associated features that represent the clues and hints that have been scattered about. As most people reading this book know, autism has many different presentations and one often hears the statement, "if you know one person with autism, you know one person with autism." Following this section, we will discuss what we know about autism and current theories on its origins, but more importantly we will discuss what we don't know.

The next part of this book requires the reader to put on an abstract thinking cap. We will consider what typically happens at age one to two that creates our adult, human ability to think _about_ the world around us, drawing on a number of theorist's ideas. There are a number of alternate terms to explain this concept, but the main idea is duality: object and symbol of the object, real and imagined reality, thinking and thinking about thinking. The relevance of these concepts will become apparent as we move on to research on meta-cognition and theory of mind (ToM), but the centerpiece of this book is something that typically is not done: we will expand one theorist's ideas and make full use of what the psychoanalytic community has to offer. With this understanding, we will consider the many ways in which developmental psychoanalytic processes might be affected, resulting, at times, in the outcome of autism. One area we will discuss is the role of cultural trends in creating the increasing numbers of persons with autism. Finally, we will take all of this learning and try to decide where we might go from here. I know this agenda sounds like a lot to get through and it is, but there is no simple way to understand or explain autism. There is no known gene or single environmental toxin that has been identified as causal. Instead, we need to use what we have and what we know to figure out autism, and the symptoms themselves can begin to illuminate why we as clinicians, parents, and researchers face such a daunting task.

The Core Symptoms

Many journal articles or chapters on autism begin the same way. Either they mention Kanner's (1943) paper which is mainly a collection of case studies, or they discuss the three main criteria that create the autism diagnosis. These three main criteria are often drawn from the Diagnostic and Statistical Manual of Mental Disorders (DSM-IV-TR), which lists autism as one of the pervasive developmental disorders (PDD). As such, autism is a lifelong disorder where the symptoms are present before age 3, and therefore it is usually diagnosed in infancy or childhood. It is marked by impairments in 1) social interactions and 2) communication, as well as 3) a restricted set of interests or repetitive behaviors. Such broad criteria can, as one would suspect, be expressed in many different ways, so fortunately the DSM provides additional information to assist clinicians. For example, social interaction impairments can affect a wide range of behaviors which change as the child ages. As an infant or young child, there may be impairments in eye-gaze, poor understanding of facial expressions, and a lack of shared enjoyment. Young children with autism will not show or bring things to others, engage in joint attention, or initiate/respond to social overtures. They may use others as "tools" in play (including unusual use of another's body or body part), and interact with disinterest, as if no one was even around them. As an older child, the person with autism additionally has difficulty with social conventions, empathy, showing insight into his or her emotions, and will not generally seek peer-related, shared enjoyment with others. This child may prefer solitary activities and have little conceptualization of (or concern for) the needs, joys, or distress of others. In essence, the autistic child is, as the name suggests conceptually, within and the same as the "self," alone in a world of others.

The DSM likewise has a number of descriptors for the communication domain. Persons with autism may not be at all able to speak, may have some speech or some form of speech delay, or can have full speech but be basically unable to sustain a reasonable conversation with another person. Delays can take the form of idiosyncratic language, limited gesturing, unusual intonation or rhythm, or even repetitive use of meaningless or "heard" language, such as books, commercials, or songs. In terms of understanding language there is a wide range of abilities, but jokes and humor are particularly difficult for some reason, and communicative play is often out of context or described as "mechanical." Similar to the social impairments, communication impairments are not always simply a delay or absence of language. Instead, these impairments take on a particular form or flavor that relates to the curious nature of autism. What I mean by this is that when speech is present, it is impaired in relation to *another person*; the person with autism cannot perceive the other person's interest or role in a mutual conversation, and has no interest in learning to create normal speech patterns. Further, beyond not understanding statements or questions, he or she has difficulty with *humor*, which interestingly involves simultaneous (or dual) comprehension of multiple meanings or words or situations. And note that similar to the socialization domain where people are identified as "tools," communication for the person with autism is described as "mechanical." As a group then, we could begin to conceive of autism as a conceptual absence of other people. And in its place, the person with autism simply sees another "thing."

Finally, the DSM discusses the third set of criteria for an autism diagnosis, restricted and repetitive patterns of behavior. Persons with autism may inflexibly focus on one particular topic with intensity, insist on performing meaningless routines or motor mannerisms, or they may have a persistent pre-occupation with "parts of objects." This leg of the autism triad of symptoms can be present in as many forms as the communication domain, and is often compared to behaviors associated with obsessive-compulsive disorder (OCD). Persons with autism may line items up, insist on a particular order to various elements in the environment, or repetitively play with the same item or watch the same video clip over and over. Any interruption in these various routines, rituals, or movements can at times lead to intense distress, far beyond what would normally be expected, or some persons with autism have no response at all to interruption of routines. They simply move on to the next item or activity of interest. Interestingly, the DSM notes that there may be a pre-occupation with "parts of objects," a fascination with movement of objects, or an intense attachment to an "inanimate object." As with the socialization and communication domains, even these clearly identified, standard, and accepted diagnostic criteria suggest some special relationship to the things in the world around the person with autism. Whether the people in this world are "tools," communicative play is "mechanical," or parts of objects are more interesting than the whole thing, there is a pervasive difference between typically developing persons and persons with autism: everything is a "thing," and for that child there has never been an "other." This may seem unusual or even benign to the reader, but as we shall see, it is the early awareness of another person as a person (not an inanimate object) that allows normal thinking to develop. Again we see that autism is aptly named; self, same self, and only a singular self exists.

While we can begin to get an idea of what autism is by examining these standard criteria, it is the associated symptoms that provide important clues as to the nature of autism. These associated symptoms don't seem to fit nicely into the standard autism triad. One example is impaired "awareness" which is typically considered related to socialization. However, this component extends beyond a domain identified by how one person interacts with another, and seems to suggest that persons with autism may or may not even know that others in the environment exist. So when a person with autism is in a group of people, how are those other people perceived? Are people perceived as moveable, animated objects? If so, how does one explain some children with autism's apparent pleasure at seeing the parent? Another example, this one typically in the communication domain, is "limited make-believe play" which is diagnostically wedged between idiosyncratic language and abnormal speech intonation. What does make-believe or imagination-based play have to do with communication and speech development? It is as if there were a collection of symptoms given to the creators of this diagnostic category, and one way or another, they had to make them fit; a difficult task indeed. They do not in fact go together easily in the categories identified, mainly because we have a very limited understanding of what autism is and where it comes from, so the categories themselves are most likely misleading. Because practitioners are unable to draw upon a coherent theory that encompasses the myriad categories and factors and creates a diagnostic framework, we are left to our own devices as to how to best capture the many complex and curious signs of autism.

Further associated symptoms of autism add to our already almost bizarre listing of criteria. Uneven cognitive skills, various behavioral challenges such as impulsive aggression or tantrums, odd responses to sensory stimulation, and abnormalities of mood are all commonly present. The person with autism may not fear what they should fear, or may be excessively fearful about seemingly innocuous elements in the environment. They may have unusual eating or sleeping habits, and it is not unusual to see a variety of self-injurious behaviors, or what clinicians refer to as "SIB." These behaviors can take many forms, including finger-or wrist-biting, head-hitting, eye-poking, and many others. This grouping of behavioral symptoms are some of the most difficult to understand and disturbing features of autism, and they are often difficult to stop or at least reduce. One of the more effective approaches to addressing SIB (as well as many other behavioral challenges) is to determine the true reason for, or function of, the behavior, a process known as functional behavioral analysis (FBA). However, a popular outcome of this process is the finding that the function is not to obtain something or avoid something, but rather "sensory." This means that the person with autism is simply seeking out or *enjoying* the sensory stimulation associated with the behavior. In addition to the other symptoms listed, how do we integrate the apparent enjoyment of self-induced pain or mutilation? And because it is neither socialization nor communication (usually), is it appropriate to consider this a repetitive behavior? While it certainly is repetitive, SIB seems conceptually different from lining up pencils or watching a video repeatedly. As perplexing and frustrating as this is, this fact gives us another clue into the origins of autism and as such is one of the many symptoms that a comprehensive theory of autism needs to be able to accommodate.

A number of other researchers have added even further to the list of features associated with a diagnosis of autism. Courchesne et al. (1990) for example, note that children with autism do not imitate others, and typically do not take turns or share attention with others. They prefer solitary play and may appear disinterested in the behaviors and actions of others. In the communication domain, these researchers suggest that some additional features include echolalic speech (repeating back the last thing that one hears), and the unusual presence of pronoun reversal. In pronoun reversal, "you" is often or always stated instead of "I," which is another seemingly bizarre and unrelated symptom that is, at the same time, another hint as to the nature of autism. In a related vein, persons with autism often apply a concrete, literal interpretation of phrases and metaphors. For example, if you said something like "we will put that idea in our back pocket," that is exactly where the person with autism would look. Interestingly, much like some forms of humor, metaphors such as these again require simultaneous comprehension of two meanings, the literal one and the conceptual one. When one begins to think more along these abstract lines in considering the nature of autism, it almost begins to make sense in a curious and vague sort of way.

Returning for a moment to pronoun reversal, this symptom has received a notable amount of research in past years, and is a good example of the heterogeneity of the disorder. In a recent article, Hobson and his colleagues (Hobson, Lee and Hobson, 2010) reviewed research that suggests highly varied presentations of pronoun reversal in terms of frequency. One research article reviewed reported 17 out of 25 (nearly 70%) children with autism displaying this feature, while in other articles reviewed, a mere 12% of participants reversed pronouns. This wide span of results that is commonly found in autism research, most likely stems from the heterogeneity of the autism diagnosis, hence the term "autism spectrum disorder," or "ASD." As we have noted, an autism diagnosis can include high or low intelligence, speech or no speech, challenging behaviors or no challenging behaviors, some attention to others or none, and the list goes on. While there is no actual ASD diagnostic category or any "high" or "low" functioning designations, those a researcher selects as his or her participants can vary widely and the product will still be considered research on persons diagnosed with autism. The diagnostic criteria are simply so broad that the variety of diagnostic triad combinations are seemingly endless. This of course can affect the results of any given research study, and unfortunately, while persons with more severe presentations of the disorder might be considered the neediest, persons with less pronounced or severe presentations are often those included in research for obvious reasons.

So to summarize what we know so far, there are a minimally coherent and homogenous group of standard diagnostic features, further associated features that only add to the complexity of this disorder, and research based on highly varied sets of participants. To complicate the picture further, different features of autism are present at different ages and then change across the lifespan. While this fact might seem to add to the confusion already created, it is again a clue as to the source and evolution of autism, and something that needs to be addressed in a comprehensive theory. We have mainly been discussing the diagnostic behaviors that constitute a childhood or adolescent picture of autism, but also note that in early infancy, parents often report extremes of temperament, poor eye contact, and a lack of response to play attempts (Zwaigenbaum et al., 2005). Infants later diagnosed with autism typically don't socially smile, lack facial expression, do not respond to their name being called, and do not orient to faces. These young infants lack spontaneous imitation, and can have abnormal muscle tone. Zwaigenbaum further suggested that it wasn't until 12 months of age or older that an autism diagnosis could be predicted; behaviors at age 6 months simply did not predict a later diagnosis. Again, just to put 'in your back pocket' for later use, these researchers' predictive behaviors (in addition to those already listed) included a passive early temperament followed by later, extreme distress reactions, and poor visual tracking associated with an increasing inability to disengage from visual stimuli. Typically developing infants on the other hand, are more and more able to disengage quickly from a visually perceived object in the environment. Simply put, Zwaigenbaum found that very young infants who were later diagnosed with autism did not actively engage with their environment in a number of ways. While this may sound somewhat harmless and in many situations may, in fact, be harmless, such non-activity was associated with serious problems shortly thereafter. Further, these young infants chose or preferred to look at one thing and then kept looking at it, and they preferred *non-social* stimuli and remained fixated on such stimuli even when there were other good things to pay attention to (as a typically developing child would). Notice again the interest in objects rather than people.

There are literally hundreds of chapters and articles that further detail the early features of autism, and researchers continue to work to identify exactly how we might better spot the disorder in its formative stages. A discussion of these many writings is beyond the scope of this chapter, but our goal here is to simply outline how unusual, complex, varied, and perplexing a fuller description of autism can be. You might have a sense that these symptoms do go together is some way, although right now it is difficult to figure out exactly how. There seems to be a theme of sorts, a central idea that we can't as yet put our finger on. At this point perhaps, all we can say is that there may be something central here about how other people are understood or perceived, and there is confusion about how they are different from inanimate objects in the environment. There is some sort of early preference for inanimate objects that must be linked to an expanding network of associated symptoms. But that framework seems like a tangled web of unrelated or at best, loosely related symptoms. What is happening early in life? How does autism result? And how could something as basic as impaired early eye gaze result in a disorder that includes symptoms as obscure as not being able to understand a joke? These are difficult questions but it seems clear that practitioners and parents alike would benefit from a coherent and encompassing theory of autism; one that accounts for both early and later symptoms, as well as ties together most of the apparently core and associated symptoms. I hope to put forth a thesis towards such a theory in this book.

Chapter 2: What We Know About Genes, Environment, Treatment, and Typical Early Development

The pathogenesis of autism is largely unknown (Bodfish, 2004), but we do know a little about prevalence, and the role of both genetics and environment. Unfortunately, what we know does not make much sense to researchers as yet. It will probably come as no surprise to anyone reading this that the number of documented cases of autism has been increasing steadily over the past 20 years. No one really knows whether this is the result of an actual increase in rates or simply better/more inclusive identification, but in 1994 the rate was approximately 3.5 in 10,000, or .00035% (APA, 2000). By 2009, the rate of children diagnosed with autism had risen to an estimated 1% of children ages 3 to 17 (Kogan et al., 2009), and no one knows the reason for the apparent increase. We do know that this disorder is found four times more frequently in males than in females, which in itself suggests a genetic origin. Further support for a genetic link comes from the fact that research on the risk of recurrence in a (genetically similar) sibling ranges between 3 and 8% (Szatmari et al., 1998). However, concordance rates in monozygotic twins (genetically identical siblings) are less than 100% (Santangelo and Tsatsanis, 2006) which instead supports the role of environmental factors. Simply put, despite a desperate search, there is no known single biological marker or gene that is responsible for the expression of autism. Although it is demonstrated very early in life, unlike Down Syndrome or Fragile X Syndrome, autism is clearly a combination of genetic _and_ environmental factors which complicates the situation dramatically. What types of genes contribute to the emergence of autism and how? What environmental factors are central? And how do these two factors combine so early in life to result in such a pervasive and debilitating disorder?

Before we move on to other research on genetics, it is important to note something in the Szatmari et al. (1998) article that is usually not highlighted because it is not clearly understood. In fact, it makes a complex situation even more complex. The article discusses much about the genetics of autism, mainly by summarizing twin studies. There are not a lot of twins with autism, so even a few studies with such a population are considered important and key in trying to understand this disorder. In Szatmari's summary tables, the reader will find information on monozygotic twins and dyzigotic twins, who have respectively, 100% and 50% (on average by descent, as with siblings) identical genetic material. There are four such studies listed, and the concordance rates for monozygotic twins ranges from 36% to 95%, with an average of 73%. This means that on average, if you have the exact same genetic material, you have a 3 out of 4 chance of developing autism. In these same studies, the concordance rates for dyzigotic twins are also listed, and with an average of 50% of the same genetic material by descent, one would expect concordance rates in the 20% to 50% range. However, what are actually listed are extremely _low_ concordance rates in these types of twins: 0% in three of the four studies listed and 23% in the last study. Out of a total of 48 pairs of dyzigotic twins, only four found both children developing autism. As one would expect, this is about the same overall concordance percentage (8%) as non-twin siblings when you average all the research findings, and the one study that found the highest concordance rate at 23% is the one criticized due to nonsystematic sampling. All of the rest of the studies showed 0% concordance rates. This complicated picture may suggest that autism is a "whole person" (generally speaking) disorder. It may suggest that the roots of autism are found in a process that draws from not one, but many of the complex and pervasive sources of our human experience. Further, this finding is another fact that we will put in our back pocket, which seems to be filling with a number of interesting clues as to the origins of autism.

Santangelo and Tsatsanis (2006) carefully stated, "It is expected that several genes are involved that, in combination, give rise to an increased vulnerability to autism" (p.77). Researchers have found perhaps 10 to 15 (or more) genetic areas that may play key roles (the 15q11-q13 region has been found to be the most common location of chromosomal abnormalities in persons with autism), but it is disheartening to realize that even positive findings of genetic commonalities only account for about 8% of persons diagnosed with the disorder. One way to hypothesize a stronger role of genes is to use terms such as the ones noted in the quote above: "in combination" and "vulnerability," for example. Such terms suggest that we have been too limited in our single-gene, single-region, or absolute 'gene X = autism' search; perhaps we need to extend our search to multiple *combinations*. Or, perhaps there are complex combinations of genes that make us *vulnerable* to an even wider variety of environmental factors. But at this point, haven't we moved into what we know about many psychological disorders? Couldn't we say the same thing about schizophrenia or depression? Although these are typically seen later in life, aren't disorders such as these likely to result from complex combinations of genetic codes that open the door to an array of environmental influences that result in the disorder? The answer to this is a resounding 'yes,' in that there are genetic similarities in persons with these disorders, yet not everyone with these similar codes develops the disorders listed.

But the _early_ emergence of autism as compared to other psychological disorders does pose a special challenge because there is so little time for environment to play its supposed role. One way of addressing this challenge is to suggest that the source of "environmental influence" is not an event or experience, but rather a "toxin" that exploits a genetic mutation early in life and/or causes some of the known abnormal brain development (e.g., Bauman and Kemper, 2003). For example, at the 2008 International Meeting for Autism Research (IMFAR), Brenda Eskenazi and Eric Roberts reported on a longitudinal study called "CHAMACOS." In this study, these researchers found that a mutation of a gene responsible for detoxification of pesticides may have contributed to the emergence of PDD. Not all of the children exposed to pesticides developed PDD, but the ones who did were genetically vulnerable. Beyond toxins such as pesticides, other environmental substances such as heavy metals, infections, and air pollution have been suggested to contribute to the "chronic pathophysiology of neuroinflammation and oxidative stress" (Herbert, 2005) of autism, yet not one of them has been scientifically proven to be causal. In essence, we are left with a conclusion that most would consider a bit obvious and of little practical value in trying to understand autism: beyond more males developing the disorder than females and concordance rates being higher in monozygotic twins as compared to dizygotic, all we know of genetics and autism is that there are a few regions of common genetic anomalies present in about 8% of the autism population. These anomalies may or may not create a vague vulnerability to any number of environmental substances or influences, but none have been scientifically found to actually be consistently causal. As Szatmari et al. (1998) note when they consider autism similar in etiology to schizophrenia or bipolar disorder, "No evidence for Mendelian subforms exist and each genetic locus appears to provide only a relatively small proportion of the increased risk to the disorder" (p.365). Not only does this tell us very little about where autism comes from (except that genetic risk seems to come from just about everywhere on our DNA), but what about the other 92% of people with autism?

So if both the genetic and environmental toxin approaches leave us wanting in terms of a satisfactory explanation as to the origins of autism, are there psychological theories? There are, and these include a variety of ideas including Baron-Cohen's Theory of Mind (ToM) deficit theory, Norman and Shallice's executive function theory, and Frith's central coherence theory. A full discussion is beyond the scope of this book, but the concepts are basically that autism derives from an inability to understand the thinking and perspectives of others, impairment in early development of the main cognitive processes, or a limited ability to understand context or see the "big picture," respectively. Each has impressive attributes or ideas, but each also leaves the reader wanting something more.

Effective Treatment

Perhaps exploring why certain types of interventions are effective in treating autism might be more illuminating than searching for genetic or environmental causes. There have been volumes written on this topic, but because we know autism is expressed early in infancy and it is only during infancy that intense treatment can sometimes affect core and not only associated symptoms, we will focus here on interventions employed during early childhood. Specifically, while many techniques have been shown to affect established symptoms of autism in later childhood, adolescence, and even adulthood (picture exchange/communication systems, medications, social scripts, daily schedule systems, functional behavior analysis, applied behavior analysis procedures, etc.), it is only during infancy that distinct alterations can perhaps be made in foundational areas and indicators such as cognitive development and educational placement. One of the first research studies that showed significant core improvements was conducted by Lovaas (1987). This researcher worked with 19 children with autism who were approximately 3.5 years of age or under, and he exposed them to two years or more of treatment that averaged 40 hours per week. It was reported that nearly 90% of the children in the experimental group achieved significant intellectual and educational gains, and that these gains were maintained years later. Despite some methodological flaws and an inability (so far) for other researchers to fully replicate these enormous gains, versions of the interventions used by Lovaas (which were all based on the principles of applied behavior analysis (ABA)) continue today to be the preferred method of intervention for children with autism. This is due to generally supportive follow-up research (e.g., Frea & McNervey, 2008).

So what actually happened during treatment in the Lovaas study, and what types of ABA interventions are used today? Early treatment models used a "discrete trial" methodology, along with ignoring, removing reinforcement for, or punishing (with a moderate slap on the thigh) non-desired behaviors (which is not generally considered appropriate or necessary today). For the discrete trial goals, a specific behavioral target was identified and modified by gaining the child's attention, giving a discrete instruction, and then reinforcing the correct response or providing any number of correction procedures for non-correct responses. This process was repeated in massed trials, and then when a measured behavioral goal was attained, a new one was put in place. Behavioral targets were individualized based on that child's particular needs and functioning levels, and targets could include anything from imitation skills, to receptive and expressive language skills, to pre-academic or daily living skills. Such "drills" of skill sets typically became more and more complex, and previously learned behaviors were reviewed periodically so no skill sets were lost. Treatment today often continues to employ this discrete trial approach with explicit teaching of additional skills such as joint attention, turn-taking, or interactive play, having sessions administered by both clinicians and parents throughout the day. However, there are a number of additional therapeutic elements that have also been found to be key in effecting a change.

Associated ABA techniques are commonly added as indicated to augment discrete trial teaching. For example, token systems can be used to reinforce desired behaviors, and functional behavior analysis can be used to help minimize inappropriate behaviors. Incidental teaching reinforces skills and behaviors outside of the discrete trial dyad, and parents take part in specialized training so that intervention can take place throughout the day. Various other ABA-derived techniques are integrated into programs such as visual schedules which provide a clear plan as to what is happening next, picture exchange communication systems allow expression of wants and needs in the absence of speech, or predictable routines and environmental structure. Rogers and Vismara (2008) note many of these interventions as components of treatment models described as "probably efficacious," the popular versions of which are Pivotal Response Training (PRT), and the Denver Model. These models elaborate on one element of treatment or another. PRT for example, uses a combined developmental and ABA perspective to increase a child's desire to learn skills related to imitation, language, and play. For the PRT therapist, the "pivotal" areas are those that when targeted, improve other related areas that were not necessarily targeted. Examples of pivotal areas include motivation, responsiveness to cue, empathy, and others (Koegel & Koegel, 2006). So, to improve early labeling and requesting, the PRT therapist might affect motivation by creating obstacle situations that serve to elicit communication attempts, and at the same time modeling appropriate prompts for the infant. Similarly, the Denver model employs selected teaching techniques within the framework of an interpersonal relationship. But it is the *one-on-one engagement and human interaction* that is often the main focus, and the scientific and systematic data-based decision-making that form the unique centerpieces of many of these effective forms of treatment.

For a child starting treatment, a focus is usually on the basic behaviors noted above that are oftentimes missing or minimal for the child with autism. For example, attending to social stimuli such as responding to one's name being called, orienting to attempts by others to engage in joint attention, and basic imitation are common places to start. While these can be addressed in a discrete trial format and often are, it is the incidental teaching in more naturalistic settings that allows skills to be generalized. Further, combining naturalistic and play-based teaching strategies in addition to discrete trial teaching makes skill acquisition more likely to become part of the child's spontaneous, functional communication. But regardless of the discrete trial or play-focused format, what is always happening in these interactions? One key feature is obvious, yet it must be clearly identified for our purposes: all of the most effective forms of intervention require another person, whether it is a teacher, parent, or clinician. These interventions can't be administered effectively in any other way, and there is no current form of effective treatment for autism that does not involve someone else being present, gaining the child's attention, establishing eye-contact, and then baiting the environment, providing reinforcement, or correcting a behavioral response in a rapid, planned, and repeated manner. The learning theory portion of this treatment equation should not come as a surprise because interventions based on these principles have been proven effective for the past 60 years; it is the human contact element that is interesting. No video, no self-management, no toys, no Skinnerian reinforcement machine, and no set of physical surroundings will do the trick. And it is not simply that there is a person present, but the amount or duration of that person's presence seems to make the difference between effective and non-effective treatment. While the 40 hours used by Lovaas may no longer be the essential number, 15 to 25 hours of intensive treatment (accompanied by trained, parent engagement at other times) is not currently considered excessive by any means. Simply put, treatment needs a person for progress to take place.

In summary, while there is clearly a heritable component to autism, genetics alone do not tell the whole story and any genetically significant areas are likely spread across vast amounts of genetic material. Our best explanation at this point in time is that there may be a small subset of children with autism that have any one of a number of chromosomal anomalies, and these anomalies may have put these children at risk under certain environmental conditions. But because there is a vast majority of other children with autism *without* these genetic anomalies, we must conclude that 1) we simply have not as yet found the responsible genetic marker, 2) there are environmental substances or influences at play in the creation of autism not yet identified, and/or 3) beyond the 8% of children with the known genetic anomalies, there are a variety of "soft" predispositions to developing autism that are not clearly identifiable in one's genetic make-up. What I am suggesting by this last item is that there remains the possibility that there may be a typically male temperament (which is not a new idea and will be returned to at a later time), set of traits, type of general approach to the world or type of "being" that is a result of and caused by many bits of the whole of our genetic endowment.

All infants have of course, certain temperaments, and we will note that such combinations of qualities are not evidenced in any specific genetic pattern or region.   For example, any given infant might be generally irritable, passive, happy, or agreeable, yet you won't find a set of genetic markers where these qualities came from. But for autism, what would such a "quality" be and how could it interact with the environment so early to cause such pervasive damage?   While it seems obvious in retrospect, looking for a gene or responsible set of genes for autism presumes that this disorder is a singular, coherent "thing" that unfolds like eye color, and clearly it is not. If only it were so simple! Similarly, there is no known substance or environmental influence that causes autism, which suggests that this is also not solely an environmentally induced problem. It may be something in the middle, something partially genetic and partially environmentally induced.   It must be something pervasive across the genetic code, and a quality that is present and active very early in development. Interestingly though, if an infant spends 20 to 40 hours per week being encouraged to pay attention to another person in a planned and intensive manner, sometimes the very core symptoms or foundational cognitive skills can be affected.   In certain cases, this type of intensive, planned, human engagement has even been reported to lead to cases of "recovery."

Typical Early Development
We have enough information now to begin thinking about what a reasonable and logical theory of autism might look like. One possibility is that in the majority of cases, autism results from genetically "softer" infantile traits, preferences, or ways of being that

collide with an important, early developmental process and/or environmental element, causing the infant to veer off of some aspect of normal developmental trajectory. Although many aspects of the young child are developing in the first year of life, I am going to add this to our hypothesis that it is the *very process of thinking* that is affected which, as I will show, accounts for nearly all of the symptoms of autism. This is by no means a new idea, but how it happens and what is happening has not been clearly identified in a manner that does all the things a comprehensive or useful theory needs to do. Of course, no infant comes into the world with adult thinking capabilities; these form over time and are a function of a developmental sequence that takes place in the context of a (hopefully) active, engaging, and appropriately stimulating environment. We know that without this stimulation, devastating damage is likely. Although "thinking" is a broad term, since we know that autism emerges by the second year, it follows that we must look at what aspects of thinking are forming before and during this early period. To do this, we need to know what is happening with typically developing infants with regard to their ability to think in both year one and year two. And it turns out that this is a particularly interesting time of development. (For the section that follows, I would like to acknowledge Jennifer Van Reet who authored much of the corresponding information in our 2011 article.)

While we know that newborns clearly can't and don't think like adults, it is difficult to conceive of what the mental world of a newborn might be like. Years ago, a child was considered a "tabula rasa" or blank slate, ready and waiting to be filled with information from the outside world. But a child does not come into the world without any thinking abilities; quite the contrary. Research has shown that even a fetus in the third trimester can become accustomed or "habituate" to a sound (Kisilevsky et al., 1999), and newborns can recognize sounds experienced in utero (DeCasper and Spence, 1986). These facts suggest that even before birth, there is the capability of even a fetus or newborn somehow "knowing" something. Granted, this "knowing" is usually a primitive form of simple recognition. Being able to "recognize" is often considered one of the most basic behaviors that signifies thinking because it suggests that some type of memory or "primary representation" has been created. While this is an impressive feat, the ability to recognize is still rather unsophisticated when we compare it to the wide range of adult thinking abilities that commonly emerge.

Within 6 months of birth, the infant has typically made some impressive cognitive strides. Research has shown that by 3 months, he or she knows something about gravity (Baillergeon et al., 1992), and soon after that, there is evidence of infants recognizing simple goal-directed behavior (Woodward, 1998). While the infant clearly cannot explicitly manipulate ideas about gravity or understand actual intention, these studies do indicate precursor abilities: the infant "recognizes" that heavy objects don't usually hang in the air, and hands can be reaching for a *certain* toy. By 8 months, the typically developing infant can demonstrate "object permanence," meaning that they know an object continues to exist even if it is hidden from view (Willatts, 1984). This skill is significant, as it indicates that the infant has developed a primitive version of a skill to which we will devote much time and attention: imagination. For an infant to search for a hidden object, they must have moved slightly beyond recognition of people, objects, or patterns in a cognitive sense. Looking for something unseen suggests that the developing infant can now actually conceive of the item in a mental way. He or she is now able to "imagine" its existence and location, and hold that mental conceptualization while searching. Note that we will use the term "imagination" in its broadest sense, defined as any behavioral evidence of a generated mental image, representative symbol, or concept.

When researchers are discussing these various mental abilities, typically they use the term "primary representation" when considering recognition, and "meta-representation" when more sophisticated, imagination-based abilities are evident. We will return to these concepts later, but it is notable that shortly after object permanence surfaces, a range of social skills typically emerge prior to the first birthday. These skills are so incredible and denote such a cognitive leap that they have often been called the "9-month revolution" (Tomasello, 1999). It is at this time that we typically begin to see many of the skills, the lack of which signifies autism. Specifically, infants begin to attend to the emotional expressions of other people for important information. The "emotional stance" of other people is "taken on" by the infant (Woodard and Van Reet, 2011), and behaviors such as joint attention, increasingly deferred imitation, and pointing emerge. Shared interest in an item or event suggests that something important has happened from a cognitive perspective, and a whole world has opened up for the developing infant.

Woodard and Van Reet propose (as have others previously) that the infant has apparently gained an early version of "thinking about": the ability to "utilize an alternative perspective. They can interpret and identify with what another person is feeling, looking at, and pointing to..." (p. 216). This shift in skills and abilities has been the focus of much research because it marks that emergence of a level of thinking far beyond object permanence; now there is not only a real object and perception of the object, but a real person and perception of the mental state of that person relative to the shared perception of object! I suggest that this development is a significant "step up" on the ladder of cognitive abstraction and is imagination itself. Our central hypothesis is thus: Autism is the result of impairment in this cognitive step, and all the associated skills that flow from it as a person develops. It is one thing to know that a box of corn flakes continues to exist even if I can't see it in the cabinet. It is quite another thing to presume the mental state of another person by watching their eyes and facial expression, and then take this one step further and conceive of that mental state. Not that these two abilities are unrelated; clearly the first lends itself to the complexity of the next, which is consistent with the cascading effects noted in our hypothesis. Note for future reference that object comes first in the process of thinking development for the infant, followed by person and mental state of the person.

This new ability to share in the emotional states and internal experiences of others allows for many new social interchanges. Infants begin to point out people and objects of interest to others, rather than simply allowing others to take the lead. They seek to join in emotional exchanges during typical development, and become what Van Reet calls a true "social partner". As time goes on during the second year of development, infants build upon these new-found abilities and become able to imagine mental states that differ from their own. By 18 months they can imagine another person's desires (Repacholi and Gopnik, 1997), and actually act on these perceived, alternate mental states. It is also during this period that we see the behavior that has been the focus of many a research study on autism: pretend play. As with our primary and meta-representational concepts, we will return to pretend play later. First we need to discuss how theorists have explained how this "9-month revolution" in thinking takes place. Because it corresponds to when we see the first signs of autism, it is essential to describe what is known (or at least theorized) about this important period of development. It is also important because imagination has cascading benefits as time goes on; empathy, language, humor, and concept of self to name a few. It makes sense theoretically that these correspond in many ways to the cascading deficits that emerge in the child with autism. What we can take from this section of our discussion is that a useful and encompassing theory of autism needs to account for a combined role of genetically pervasive influence and very early environmental factors, and a preponderance of males with the disorder. A theory of autism must explain why the only effective, empirically validated interventions involve many hours of intense contact with people, and focus on processes active in the first year of development. Specifically, the same seemingly effortless changes in thinking for the typical child around the first birthday are absent in the child with autism.

Chapter 3: Explanations of the 9-month Revolution in Thinking: The Emergence of Imagination

The period of development dubbed the "9-month revolution" may bear special importance when we are considering the origins of autism for a number of reasons. First, as noted above, it signifies a monumental change in how the infant behaves and thinks, and these changes directly correspond to the pervasive, resultant abilities that comprise to the basic diagnostic indicators for autism. I will suggest that they also correspond to the "cascading" problems commonly seen as autism progresses. By this I mean that initially, delays in infant responding or joint attention may not seem so worrisome; despite being diagnostic indicators, parents are often told that such variations are normal and to simply "wait and see." But these types of behaviors relate directly not only to autism, but many adult thinking abilities and foundational concepts (such as "self") may derive from successful navigation of developmental processes during this period, and thus may be subsequently affected. In essence, I am suggesting first that <u>autism is the result of early impairment in the development of foundational, early imagination or meta-representational abilities, which has cascading effects as the child continues to develop</u>. Second, the 9-month revolution happens very early in development, making the timing match when the first signs of autism are present. And third, the infant typically moves into and through this period of development so seamlessly that there is general agreement that it has a genetic base. However, research suggests that development certainly can be affected during this period by environmental influences, such as deprivation, toxins, or non-stimulation. We will discuss theorists who have made significant contributions to our knowledge about the 9-month revolution, and consider each of their unique perspectives in turn. Understanding the mechanisms that allow for early imaginative or meta-representational thinking will be central to developing effective interventions, if our thesis is correct.

Jean Piaget

Jean Piaget was one of the great developmental theorists of our time, and one of the first to suggest that early behaviors (such as pretend play) contributed to how we think as adults. Piaget's theories were derived from close observation of children, and based on the idea that reality was constructed from incoming information drawn from the infant's continual engagement with objects and people in his environment. Piaget's developmental perspective of ever-increasing ideas and understanding depended on a core set of central concepts: schemas, assimilation, and accommodation. Schemas are sets of perceptions or ideas that are logically associated with each other, assimilation denotes the addition of information into an existing schema, and accommodation means that a schema itself needs to be adjusted to manage newly assimilated information. While these definitions appear simple, his use and application of these ideas to the various stages of development that he hypothesized become increasingly complex. Piaget's theories cover a great deal of the development of children, but we are mainly interested in what he identified as the later section of the "sensori-motor" stage since it corresponds to the latter half of an infant's first year. During this period, the infant moves from simple reflexes to "primary" and then "secondary circular reactions," where awareness of external objects increases and attempts are made to actually reproduce events (such as shaking a rattle). Further, as the infant repeatedly observes that actions lead to consistent consequences, he or she begins to combine behavior in new ways to accomplish goals, and becomes increasingly flexible and creative in behaviors. At this stage of development, the infant is able to replace trial and error behavior with behavior that he or she _knows_ will bring about certain results (Piaget, 1952).

But what did Piaget mean by "knowing"? And is it something that happens suddenly and without cause or reason, or is there a progression that leads to this ability? Piaget created an important work that speaks to these questions entitled "Play, Dreams, and Imitation in Childhood" (Piaget, 1962). Interestingly, as with all of Piaget's cited works, this book is a translation from French, and originally called "La Formation du Symbol," or "The Formation of the Symbol." In this book, Piaget focuses on the importance of the infant's early imitation abilities, and how these change to support later symbolic, mental representation. He differentiates clearly between very early imitation that is in the presence of a model, and later types of representative imitation, that can be deferred or where something can "stand for" something else. In the more primitive form of imitation, the visual and auditory perceptions in *immediate* experience allow for *immediate* imitation. In time however, the perceptions somehow become available internally, and the infant is able to support the more sophisticated, representative forms of imitation:

"It is imitation that has been interiorised as a draft for future exterior imitation, and marks the junction-point between the sensory-motor and the representative." (p.279)

How or *why* this 'interiorising' takes place is not nearly as clearly explained as *what* takes place, but continued assimilation of information via object manipulation is noted to be essential for the emergence of more sophisticated forms of mental representation. That is to say that a continued influx of sensory perceptions and explorations of the world may create a sort of framework or priming effect (this can only be presumed as no actual mechanism is proposed by Piaget) for subsequent "symbolic or imaged representation."

With this type of higher representation now active, experimentation can now take place internally rather that externally, and mental planning and prediction become possible. In Piaget's words:

"It is therefore due to representation that 'mental experience' succeeds actual experimentation and that assimilatory activity can be pursued and purified on a new plane, separate from that of immediate perception or action so properly called." (p. 351)

This mental representation ability that emerges allows for a number of other, dependent skills to develop: invention, symbolization, and deferred imitation. These all have special significance when we return to our discussion of autism, because a very different thinking component or ability is essential to support them. "Invention" is the ability to "spontaneously" reorganize (accommodate) information in a rapid manner; in other words, to come up with new ways of thinking quickly and efficiently. "Symbolization" allows for one thing to represent another, and is most obviously necessary for the development of language. And finally, "deferred imitation" allows infants to display behaviors seen days earlier, a skill quite different from a younger infant's immediate mimicking of parental movement.

This development of symbolic or imaged representation formed the basis for not only language development, but also pretend play. For Piaget, pretend play was conceptually different from objective thought, in that it provided a "symbolic transposition which subjects things to the child's activity, without rules or limitations" (p. 87). He suggested that pretend play was nearly "pure assimilation," connecting one thing to another and, interestingly from a psychoanalytic perspective, "everything to the ego." So the progression began earlier in year one: early, immediate perceptions and imitation provided the groundwork for internalization or 'interiorisation," which then supported and primed cognition for more sophisticated, symbolic, representational thought. This, in turn, supported a range of skills including deferred imitation, as well as reality-based and more "ludic" forms of pretend play. Importantly from Piaget's perspective, such were the seeds of intelligence and creative thinking:

"This is why play is accompanied by a feeling of freedom and is the herald of art, which is the full flowering of this spontaneous creation." (p.152)

What can we say about Piaget's early description of what happens at the end of year one and into year two? How can we conceptualize what important and unique change has taken place? I will suggest that this shift from primary recognition and imitation of immediate experience to mental representation is analogous to being given a type of cognitive "workspace." In other words, it creates a secondary component of thinking where we can "set down" the objects we perceive or ideas we have and think *about* them, rather than only knowing of them in immediate experience. This is a central idea that the reader must grasp, because as we consider mental representation in ever-expanding forms, from object to less tangible concepts, we are actually talking about "imagination" as we have defined it. Because you as the reader are an adult thinker who uses this secondary workspace continually and without effort, it may be somewhat difficult to conceive of life without it. But imagine (yes, you have to use the same ability I am suggesting emerges, to consider what it is like not to have it!) that objects did not continue to exist when you could not see them. Imagine not having a cognitive "space" to problem-solve, or maintain a word or phrase's meaning alternate to its literal one. Imagine your immediate experience engulfing the entirety of your cognitive functioning, with no optional "holding" area for reflection or cognitive manipulation. Imagine you could not employ the use of symbols or language. And imagine having no cognitive space to conceive of the mental states, emotions, or intentions of other people; people would be a curious enigma, not much different from everyday objects. I am getting a bit ahead of myself in our discussion, but the importance of these early foundational skills quickly becomes apparent. These ideas may suggest in part, what the mental experience might be like for the person with autism, culminating in what we will see is a non-existent, distorted, or fractured sense or image of self.

Michael Tomasello

By employing concepts such as assimilation and accommodation, Piaget was able to hypothesize how an infant's developmental process proceeded as a result of his or her information-producing, active engagement with objects and people in the world. However, as noted previously, more recent research has shown that the infant comes into the world equipped with certain cognitive abilities that precede even the earliest manipulation of objects. Michael Tomasello has researched the manner in which these abilities emerge, and has shown how they correspond to early primate patterns (Tomasello, 1999). Further, he has proposed that there are a number of behaviors that emerge shortly after birth that demonstrate how human infants are distinctly different from their primate relatives. First, in the initial few months of life, infants engage in "protoconversations" with caregivers, which are shared visual, tactile, and vocal interchanges where emotional states appear to be communicated. Second, as was mentioned by Piaget, human infants as early as three months will immediately imitate head and mouth movements modeled for them, and by six months will even modify their behavior to match that of the model. Interestingly (and for later discussion), Tomasello suggests that these early forms of imitation indicates a "very deep identification process" (p.60).

While some might suggest that similar forms of these behaviors exist in the primate world, we turn to what Tomasello (and others) has dubbed the 9-month revolution. If there was any doubt that humans were cognitively different from primates at six months, this doubt is certainly erased by skills shown at nine months. During the same period late in the first year when Piaget suggested "interiorisation" or mental representation, Tomasello likewise notes that behaviors emerge which suggest a very different and uniquely human way of thinking. Specifically, in the months prior to the first birthday, human infants begin to engage in behaviors that include joint-attention, gaze following, and social referencing of the parent. These "referential" behaviors are soon followed by the related behaviors of pointing and showing, and as a group, come about in very close developmental synchrony. Tomasello suggests that these conceptually unique types of behaviors derive from a "dawning" understanding that others, like the self, are "intentional agents." That is, the infant begins to demonstrate via these behaviors, an understanding that other people have intentional "relations" to objects similar to the infant's own. As a result, the infant can, in many ways, now share with another in experiences. What were "dyadic" interactions with either objects or people now become "triadic" in that there emerges a "referential triangle of child, adult, and the object or event" (p. 62).

But what is the underlying mechanism for these emerging, distinctly human behaviors? Why is there a "dawning" and how does it take place? Tomasello correctly notes that the absence of these behaviors is diagnostic for autism, and so it may be essential to our goal to understand the precise trigger and process for the cognitive shift that occurs. Exactly how does this miraculous realization happen? It is suggested by Tomasello that some sort of "simulation" operation takes place where the infant comes to appreciate that others are "like me," and un-like any relationship the infant has with inanimate objects. In other words, as the infant becomes increasingly aware of his own intentions toward objects, he assigns the same internal events to other people. As the infant understands the self more and more, so does he or she understand others because they "simulate" the supposed internal workings of the other person. While there are similarities between these ideas and those suggested earlier by Piaget, Tomasello puts forth a much more specific mechanism or process, or does he?

Tomasello hypothesizes that 1) the infant becomes aware of his or her own intent toward objects in the world, and 2) sees others performing (presumably) behaviors representative of the same intent, and 3) infers that the internal, cognitive workings of other people are like the infant's own. But does this really explain the cognitive shift that has taken place? How does the infant come to be able to conceive of his or her own intent? Where does this ability to think about "intent" come from (since it is this imaginative ability that allows for the behaviors we see at nine months)? It seems that "intent" is a concept that Tomasello is running on the same explanatory "tracks" that he may be attempting to create! By this I mean that one's own or someone else's "intent" is not something that can be seen or held; it must be imagined. Again, it is the emergence of this more abstract form of imagination itself that supports the distinctly human and "triadic" behaviors of joint-attention, gaze following, and social referencing. That the infant has built upon or expanded his or her ability to imagine objects continuing to exist even though he or she can't see them, and now is able to imagine that others are "knowing," "thinking," or "intending" is the central cognitive leap that had occurred.

We use this term "imagination" broadly as we first defined it, and I would suggest that object "imagination" for example, supports object permanence, and later intent "imagination" supports the behaviors representing the 9-month revolution. Tomasello all but makes this essential point:

"...the child simply sees or imagines the goal-state the other person is intending to achieve in much the same way that she would imagine it for herself, and she then just sees the other person's behavior as directed toward that goal in much the same way the she sees her own." (p.76)

So our central question here becomes, what mechanism allows for the emergence of imagination capacities? This is a core question, but unfortunately as we as seen, Tomasello's "like me" simulation concept does little to provide us with answers. Perhaps however, this was not his purpose; the "like me" simulation was suggested to explain triadic *behaviors*, not the cognitive structures supporting them. However, Tomasello's writings in some ways, do suggest a cognitive substrate. He discusses more complex imitative acts later in his writings, the emergence of symbolic play, and perhaps one of the most complex representations of imagination, a concept of self. In his own words:

"...the human understanding of others as intentional beings makes its initial appearance around nine months of age, but its real power becomes apparent only gradually as children actively employ the cultural tools that this understanding *enables them to master*..." (italics added) (p. 56)

Before we move on to other theorists who have attempted to tackle the cognitive shift of the nine-month old infant, we need to mention two items related to our current discussion of Michael Tomasello's work. First, he uses a term that will certainly come up again in this book: "aboutness." Tomasello suggests that prior to nine months of age, infants may perceive other people as animate objects that have the ability to "make things happen in some global way." But when an infant nine to twelve months begins to understand and assign "intent," he or she is now demonstrating this "aboutness" in that, presumably, the infant is not only knowing, but now knowing "about." Similarly, we might say that we know a ball as an object if we see it, but it is something very different to say that we know "about" it. "Aboutness" suggests that we know perhaps physical properties of the ball, what it does or can do, that it exists even though we can't see it right now, and perhaps what it is not. When we switch from "knowing" to "aboutness," increasingly abstract imaginative capacities not only become helpful, they become essential.

The second item related to Tomasello that I would like to mention before we move on, has to do with the term "triadic." Tomasello and others use the term to explain the emergence of the referential "triangle" of child, other, and object, and it is contrasted with "dyadic." As we delve into this topic further, we will need a term to represent the imaginative capacities that come "online" at nine months of age, and fortunately or unfortunately (depending on how you look at it), "triadic" fits the bill nicely. As we progress, the "triad" we discuss will not be child, other, and object, but rather child, other or object, and the thinking or imagination that holds the other or the object. For example, dyadic, "here and now" thinking of the five-month old infant consists of child and other, or child and object. What exists is what is present at that moment in time. At nine months of age however, imagination allows not only the child and the object or other to exist, but adds the third element of the triangle: existence of the absent object, or intent of the other person. You might be beginning to conceive now of this imaginative ability you have and how central it is to your functioning as a person. Not to get too far ahead of ourselves, but what would life be like without it? Or what would life and your existence be like if something went very wrong at this core step in the creation of your own human thinking?

<u>Daniel Stern and Peter Fonagy</u>

The next theorist who has attempted to explain the shift in cognition that takes place is Daniel Stern, who is quite possibly one of the finest thinkers of our time. Stern (1985) takes a somewhat different view of the 9-month revolution than Tomasello, but you will notice a number of similarities, the most obvious being a "like me" concept. However, for Stern, the infant realizes the parent is *emotionally* similar, as opposed to being *cognitively* similar. In addition to the infant coming to understand that others have intent, Stern's theory adds an understanding of the caregiver's feelings.

Prior to the nine-month events previously mentioned, Stern suggests that the mother and infant are in a state of "core-relatedness." This term may sound like it is describing some type of close, relational bond between the two, but it is in fact, a basic, early, experiential sense that mother and child are physically <u>separate</u> beings. The infant is suggested to start at this point, which denotes separate affective states as well as histories. There is no understanding of the parent as having his or her own mind; rather, he or she is another thing or "agent" out in the world. The "quantum leap" that takes place toward the end of the first year of life is when the infant "gradually comes upon the momentous realization" (p. 124) that thinking can be shared with someone else. Stern acknowledges that these new abilities rest upon an entirely new set of capacities as compared to those needed for core-relatedness:

"These include the capacities for sharing a focus of attention, for attributing intentions and motives to others and apprehending them correctly, and for attributing the existence of states of feeling in others and sensing whether or not they are congruent with one's own state of feeling." (p.27)

In a state of more sophisticated, shared, or *intersubjective* relatedness, communication is achieved through gestures, facial expressions, and related social referencing. The central event taking place that accounts for this leap is fueled by affective states that are confirmed by watching the parent's emotional response; this is what Stern refers to as "inter-affectivity."

This stage is proposed by Stern to be critical to the creation of thinking and human development, and it is notable that he suggests what may occur should something go awry. In Stern's words, "At one end is psychic human membership, (and) at the other (is) psychic isolation" (p. 126). What else is autism if not psychic, and subsequent social isolation? The reader may be wondering, what mechanism does Stern use to explain the emergence of the intersubjective perspective? He suggests the concept of "affect attunement," which has not been lost on autism researchers and theorists (e.g., Dawson, 1991; Rogers, Cook, & Meryl, 2005). In fact, Dawson

(1991) has suggested that engagement in social interactions and the processing of novel and complex stimulus features necessary for affect attunement may be absent in persons with autism. The emergence of affect attunement is considered by Stern to be innate, and consists of a series of steps, beginning with the parent reading the child's feeling state accurately, and then performing an imitative behavior of that emotion. In return, the child realizes that there is affective correspondence or agreement, and finds the parent's imitative behavior enjoyable, so the reciprocal engagement continues. While this may appear to be similar to concepts such as "mirroring" or "affect matching" (and is to a degree), Stern focuses on the quality of *feeling* being shared, and less on the physical behavior itself. What is essential is a type of affective link that "can only be alluded to; it cannot be described (although poets can evoke it)" (p.27). Such words are reminiscent of Tomasello's reference to a deep, almost elusive, identification or joining with the parent.

The shift to the intersubjective stage is proposed by Stern to be crucial because it allows the infant entry into the psychological community. When the infant realizes that thinking can be shared with someone else, he or she has basically acquired "a 'theory' of separate minds" (p.124). In effect, Stern is saying that it occurs to the infant that what is going on internally matches what is going on for the other person, much like Tomasello's "like me" approach. However, the infant is not considered to be aware of any of these processes in any way that would suggest the ability to think about them in any "objectified" way. Rather this theory somehow opens the door to the psychological community by virtue of the subsequent emergence of skills: language, recall, symbolic play, and finally references to the self as an objectified entity. These skills typically emerge during the middle of the second year of life and later, and along with deferred imitation, are dependent on the need for a central skill: dual versions of reality, or the ability to imagine. The child develops the ability to represent objects not present, use words to represent objects, engage in true reality and the simulated reality of symbolic play, and both engage in behavior and represent cognitively their own execution of that same behavior. The typically developing child is able to move seamlessly between these various versions or layers of reality; he or she becomes able to think "about" objects (not just interact with them), events in time (not just the "now"), and not only who he or she and others are, but who or what they could be in an imaginary world. With time, the young child is able to conceive of the self as an object as evident through the use of pronouns, establishment of gender identity, and "acts of empathy" (p. 165).

These emerging capacities are referred to by Stern himself simply as "imagination," but ultimately allow for what you and I enjoy cognitively on a continual, moment to moment basis. This process allows for complex, sophisticated, and mature perspective-taking, perception and prediction of intentions and expectations, and imagining alternatives both real and non-real. But have we really explained a mechanism by which all of these abilities come to be, or simply created names for the capabilities that are "realized," or "come about"? Does the parent performing matching imitative emotions really explain the emergence of the ability to "think about" any better than Tomasello's infant matching the intent of others to his or her own? Regardless of what you call it, thinking about, imagination, a second layer of processing abilities, intersubjectivity, or a term we will soon encounter, "meta-representation," none of the theorists so far explain *how* it happens; they give no actual process or mechanism, but do a beautiful job of telling us *what* is happening! Before we move on to the work of Peter Hobson, we need to mention Peter Fonagy, because his theory does tweak what Stern has offered just enough to give us some sense of what a true mechanism might look like.

Much like Tomasello and Stern, Peter Fonagy and his colleagues (Fonagy, Gergely, Jurist, & Target, 2002) have suggested that similarities between the inner and outer world of the infant are at the core of the development of human cognition. Specifically, Fonagy argues that as the child expresses emotion, the parent reflects that same emotion in a "nearly, but clearly not, like me" manner. This theoretical orientation may look much like what Stern has put forth, but you will notice that it is not the "like me" concept that is central here; it is the "clearly not" portion to which we need to attend. When the parent imitates the infant's affect, Fonagy acknowledges that to the best of the parent's ability, the emotion of the infant will be "mirrored." But in reality, what the parent returns to the infant is clearly not a mirror image; it is slightly different in a number of ways. First, it is not the infant's image that the infant sees (of course), but rather someone else. In fact, it is likely to be a range of other people, because rarely does only one person interact with the child, and the instinct to mirror affect is a common one, even among the least parental of us! Second, the affect that is mirrored is likely to be an exaggerated version of the infant's and is delayed in time, so the infant expresses emotion and then slightly later sees a similar sounding and similar looking version of that emotion.

Interestingly, research tells us that infants prefer a bit of spice in their life, and will work for slightly novel stimuli to be presented. In fact, the form of mirroring or reflection described above is preferred over an exact reflection. Fonagy suggests that it is the altered parental presentation that has central value to the infant, but why? Imagine for a moment that someone has recorded your interactions at a meeting, because that person wants you to actually see how you behave. You think you are quite pleasant and cooperative at meetings, but after watching the recording, you see that in fact you are a bit pushy and need to have things go your way. Your first thought is likely to be something like, "Am I really like that?" When you ask that question, you are reflecting on yourself; you can see how the situation creates a sort of teaching environment that prompts a comparison of perceived self with real behavior. Now imagine what it must be like for an infant; these experiences are designed to prompt the very formation of the skill needed to figure them out. Fonagy calls this a "social biofeedback model" because the "nearly, but clearly not, like me" image provides a regulating or teaching environment by which the parent's affect can be internalized "through the establishment of secondary representations of the infant's primary emotion states" (p. 190). In other words, having a similar but not matching model all but forces the infant to create, activate, or "bring online" a secondary processing process to accommodate the parent's affective information.

Unlike Piaget, Tomasello, and Stern, Peter Fonagy suggests an actual mechanism by which the infant develops this capacity to "think about." Fonagy adds to our growing store of "thinking about" terms by suggesting "secondary representations," which contain the <u>parent's</u> emotional information; thus the term "internalization." Similar to Tomasello's use of the term "identification," the infant is somehow "taking in" the parent because the parent offers similar, yet slightly different versions of the infant's own feelings. In essence, the parent's ability to imagine and then imitate the emotional expression of the child is guiding the emergence of the same abilities in the infant. As with Stern, the significance of this process is acknowledged by Fonagy:

"These secondary representational structures will provide the cognitive means for assessing and attributing emotion states *to the self* that will form the basis for the infant's emerging ability to control as well as to reason *about* his dispositional emotion states." (italics added) (p. 202)

So it seems that we are a bit closer to our goal of understanding what happens early in life that forms the foundation for mature adult thinking.

In closing, Stern and Fonagy agree that emotional reflection, imitation, matching, and engagement are essential components of typical cognitive development. Both agree that these processes are foundational to the cognitive ability to form representations, think about, create non-realities, or any other term that relies on the general ability to imagine. We will turn now to how these theories have impacted research on autism; not only from the perspective of typical nine-month abilities often being impaired or absent for the child with autism, but also in terms of one of the primary and most obvious set of behaviors supported by imagination: pretend play.

Chapter 4: Imagination, Symbolism, and Pretend Play in Autism

Let's take a moment to summarize where we are in trying to better understand autism. We have discussed the standard diagnostic features of autism in the social domain such as early impairment in eye-gaze, joint attention, and shared enjoyment, which with time evolve into problems with social conventions, personal insight, and understanding the emotions of others. In the communication domain, impairments range from no speech to unusual speech to (later) poor conversation, and in the repetitive or restricted interests domain we have symptoms ranging from motor mannerisms ("hand-flapping") and a fascination with parts of objects, to an inflexible focus on one topic. Unusual symptoms that don't seem to fit anywhere in this triad of domains include things like impaired pretend play, unusual sensory responsiveness, and/or aggressive or self-injurious behaviors. For the diagnosis to be made, these symptoms need to be present before age three, and in an effort towards early identification, we know a little about young infants who were later diagnosed with autism. Specifically, it is difficult to identify a child much younger than one year of age as having autistic symptoms, but some infants with autism do show extremes in temperament, no response to social smile, and a preference for non-social stimuli. As we look back on what we have covered here, I want to point out the overall non-interest in social engagement which is rather obvious, and remind the reader about repeated, direct and indirect references that show up with regard to "objects" or "things." There is an early, general disinterest in social engagement, accompanied by not only a preference for non-social stimuli (a fancy way to say inanimate objects), but also "mechanical" communication and a tendency to use others as "tools" in interactions. In the same vein, there is a fascination with "parts of objects."

Further summarizing, we know that currently no known single gene or set of genes have been found to be causal. While there are some genetic indicators such as more males developing the disorder than females, environmental influences are also clearly evident and the responsible influences must be active in the first year of life. Treatment that has shown some effectiveness involves active, intense, and high frequency engagement with other people. This engagement focuses on increasing measured and targeted behaviors found to be lacking in the child with autism, such as eye-contact, functional communication, and attention. Further, we are interested in the behaviors that create the "9-month revolution" in thinking, not only because of the timing of this event, but also because the skills that mark this event are, in many ways, the inverse of the symptoms of autism (joint attention, attending to facial expression, shared interest, showing, etc.). Taken as a group, one way to characterize these skills is that the infant has started to "imagine" in a very broad sense of the word, or that the infant has started to be able to think "about" things. Specifically, it seems that the infant comes to imagine concrete objects (as in object permanence), and then typically moves on to more abstract things, like object function or the emotions/thinking of others, laying the essential groundwork for progressively more complex and sophisticated skills and abilities. I want to be very clear in what I am driving at:

Considered in this way, imagination, defined as the generation of mental images, representative symbols, or thinking concepts, is the skill that supports a full continuum of abilities that may be absent to varying degrees in the child with autism. These skills are primitively demonstrated early in life through image-based object permanence, and extend to imagining such things as the concept of intent or emotion of another (corresponding to the 9-month revolution behaviors). Later, these skills may provide a means for symbol-based language and imagined alternative reality of pretend play, and open the door to more sophisticated dual-thinking abilities such as empathy, shame, and the concept of self.

It may be helpful to summarize some of the imagination-based or meta-representative skills and behaviors that I am suggesting emerge early in development, and then continue to become evident in different ways as the child ages:

Proposed Indicators of Early Meta-representative or Imagination-based Skills	Typically Impaired or Absent in Autism
Object permanence	Variable
Functional object use	Yes
Response to name	Yes
Social Referencing	Yes
Pointing/use of gesture	Yes
Joint attention	Yes
Social initiation	Yes
Shared enjoyment	Yes

Later Associated Skills

Language	Variable
Recall	Yes
Deferred imitation	Yes
Use of pronouns	Yes
Shyness	Yes
Pretend/symbolic play	Variable
Concept of past and future	Variable

Associated Skills of Childhood

Perspective-taking	Yes
Theory of Mind	Yes
Acting on the desires of others	Yes
Embarrassment	Yes
Humor	Yes
Coy behavior	Yes
Lying	Yes (?)

Much Later Associated Skills

Self-reflection and insight	Yes
Object of other's critical thinking	Yes
Subtle social conventions	Yes
Concept of "self"	Yes
Problem-solving	Yes
Hypothesis creation	Yes

Finally, theories we have discussed to better understand the mechanism for the root development of what allows for such imagination include Piaget's "interiorisation," Tomasello's "intentional agent like me" perspective, Stern's "affective attunement," and Fonagy's "like me but clearly not me" idea. While each of these has its merits, all rely to a great extent on the infant simply "realizing." The theories do not provide much in terms of explanation for how the actual supporting thinking structures may be built or created, which is what we need if we are to theorize what goes awry in autism. Moreover, while each of the theorists in some manner suggests that autism is related to not successfully navigating the 9-month revolution, few have linked these formative ideas to autism as much as Peter Hobson.

In this next section we will discuss Hobson's contribution to this area, and then turn to a behavior that most everyone considers the 'holy grail' in representing imagination: pretend play. While it may be difficult for some to conceive of object permanence or joint attention as forms of imagination, few behaviors so clearly exemplify the combined image-based and concept-based forms of imagining as pretending. Not surprisingly, this behavior is typically impaired in the child with autism, and for all of these reasons has received a great deal of, and yet controversial, research attention. But first, let us discuss the work of Peter Hobson. I reviewed his work at length (Woodard & Van Reet, 2011) for a number of reasons. First, Hobson (2002) was interested in how infants shift from one way of thinking to another toward the end of the first year of development and into year two. Second, he discussed at length what could go wrong with thinking, specifically and repeatedly citing autism. Early in this work, Hobson clearly states his idea:

"Centrally and critically, autism reveals what it means to have mutual engagement with someone else. It reveals this by presenting us with the tragic picture of human beings for whom such engagement is partial or missing. The autistic child's lack of emotional connectedness with others is devastating in its own right, but also has quite startling implications for the child's ability to think. These implications are what enable us to see how thinking itself is born out of interpersonal relations." (p.5)

In his descriptions of early behavior, Hobson notes that the very young infant is typically highly attuned to the social behavior of others, and as we have noted previously, is able to imitate others and is generally interested in the faces of others. The infant typically engages easily in the mutual, emotion-laden interchanges of mother and child, but interestingly, these social behaviors are accompanied by the non-functional use of objects (e.g., banging a toy phone rather that any approximation of its intended use) and interest only in objects that are present in the infant's environment. So while there is a strong and basic emotional connection, thinking remains very dyadic, singular, and immediate.

As year two begins and then progresses, the infant starts to show the types of behavior that are indicative of what we have been calling the 9-month revolution: the infant gestures to communicate to the parent, shows items to the parent, points, and becomes more interested in (and typically consistent with) the parent's affective response to events. Hobson suggests that a clear step in thinking sophistication is now evident, but at this early stage of the cognitive progression, the infant does not yet realize that others have minds of their own. So although these behaviors as a group do not signal an infant's understanding that the other person has a mind of her own per se, there is a foundational, new form of triadic "about-ness" in thinking:

"Objects and events can be communicated about. Or, to put this another way, the infant's interactions with another person begin to have reference to the things that surround them...These events reveal that infant is no longer restricted to a focus either on an object or a person, but instead may be sensitive to a person's relation to an object." (p. 62)

In a sense, the infant is becoming more and more aware of the uniquely separate behaviors and thinking of other people as time goes on. A basic awareness of others and objects as having the potential for a relationship with each other has begun to emerge; the infant is no longer as limited to "here and now" thinking, and we see again the now familiar cognitive leap to thinking "about." But how does Hobson explain what is happening? What does he think is taking place? Hobson suggests that certain supporting behaviors such as imitation of others and assumption of their attitudes take place "automatically," and create the foundation for the later emergence of abilities such as consciously chosen perspective taking. But for now, the infant is only aware that there are others in the world with information, and the infant watches them, imitates them, and assumes their emotional reactions, because the infant is "innately equipped" to do so.

For Hobson, the next steps in how thinking develops are marked by a growing sense of self and others, language, and symbolic or pretend play. Reviewing all of these areas is beyond the scope of this book, and as noted earlier, we will focus on pretend play. It is not that language (as a form of representative symbols) or a conceptualization of self are not good examples of the ability to think about or imagination; it is simply that pretend play provides one of the best and clearest example of this, and embodies some interesting terminology that is related to concepts we have proposed, and has received research attention that may be of help in better understanding autism. Hobson discusses object substitution as one form of pretend play, which is when a child allows one thing to "stand for" another. For example, a banana "becomes" a telephone, or a rock "becomes" a car. This type of behavior suggests that the infant is now able to conceive of objects in a very different way. The infant can not only understand what the object is, but also what the object could be (but is clearly not). As pretend play progresses, the child may choose to draw in an adult to share in the pretend event. This demonstrates a real deepening of simple awareness of the psychological stance of another, in that now there is the beginning of an acknowledgment that this other person has an active mind of their own with a variety of functions and facets. The other person is now perceived as having volitional ideas, desires, and wishes of their own, and these can be real or imagined; the child can use these, reconstruct them, and integrate them into interactive, reality- or fantasy-based, spontaneous play.

Think of it! In just one year, dyadic, here-and-now thinking and interactions with objects and people have developed into the ability to think *about* them. The resulting information and understandings can, and are typically shared then with others. As year one progresses, the infant builds upon these base abilities and becomes able to depart momentarily from reality into a generated, imagined world. The infant can simultaneously maintain a concept of reality and one of non-reality, and can move seamlessly between the two. Others can become part of this world, and soon evolve into active players with imagined ideas and roles of their own. Note that for Hobson, the early base abilities are linked to and support other subsequent events as we have noted above, such as thinking about the self as a self, shyness, and embarrassment. These demonstrate the child's further cognitive extension into the ability to conceive of the self as the object of another's critical evaluation. But as far as pretend play is concerned, what is proposed by Hobson (and other theorists) about this gold-standard behavioral marker of the emergence of "about-ness" thinking needs to be compared to research. While it might look as if we are veering off-track slightly, but this is an important set of ideas that we will turn to for just a moment. We will then come back to Hobson's mechanism for how all this thinking evolution takes place.

What We Know About Imagination and Pretend Play

Few behaviors are as representative of imagination or symbolic thinking as pretend play, and the "how and why" of early pretend play has been a central question since the time of Piaget. What is the purpose of pretend play? How does it happen? How does something so apparently confusing and non-adaptive as creating a non-reality serve a child in a positive way along a developmental trajectory? As we have noted earlier, impairments in pretend play are diagnostic for autism, and even its presence in the diagnostic features is riddled with confusion. Under which domain should pretend play be subsumed? Is it a social behavior? Is it a communication behavior? What does impairment in this area mean for a child with autism? What does it tell us about what is happening internally or psychologically for this child? As early as the 1970's and continuing into the 1980's, researchers were already asking these questions. Wing, Gould, Yates, and Brierley (1977), for example, were some of the early researchers who defined functional play as the use of objects (including miniature versions of objects) as they are typically intended (a little teacup is used as one uses a teacup, or a play phone for a phone). Symbolic or pretend play (these terms are used interchangeably) in contrast, was defined as object substitution, imagining objects not present ("drinking" from a cup when no object is actually present), or imagining specific properties of an absent object. The early research generated by Wing et al. (1977) and later researchers (e.g., Mundy et al. 1986) suggested that children with autism were able to generate some pretend play, but the play was less *spontaneous and complex* compared to typically developing children. In addition, the play was much *more repetitive* (or less varied) when children with autism were compared to typically developing children.

At the time, the concepts used to explain pretend play (and then by association and extension, the concepts proposed to be impaired in autism) were "primary representations" and "meta-representations." In Leslie's (1987) theory, a primary representation was defined as a depiction of the world in an "accurate, faithful, and literal way" (p. 414); however, exactly what a primary representation was and how it differed from a perception or image or memory is not clear. There were many other authors who used this term such as Perner (1991), but they provided equally unsatisfying definitions: "A representation is something that stands in a representing relation to something else" (p. 18). It may be that Leslie simply had created another word to lay the groundwork for the dual-thinking model we have been discussing. Sure enough, Leslie subsequently suggested that during the second year of life, a "meta-representational" mechanism developed in addition to "primary representations." For Leslie, meta-representations were defined as "not representations of the world but representations of representation" (p. 417), and these versions could be altered or reconstructed. In fact, meta-representations allowed for the capacity to actively imagine, and generate a range of indefinitely reconstructable mental images or concepts. Obviously, the meta-representations deviated in fundamental ways from primary representations of the real world, at the whim of the person doing the imagining. Leslie's specific mechanism for this was that the infant developed the ability to "decouple" (that is, to separate) the primary representation from reality by creating the "meta" copy of it. The infant thus developed the ability to suspend reality and engage in pretend play by creating and manipulating the meta-, decoupled representation while at the same time leaving the primary representation of reality intact.

So Leslie theorized that autistic children are not able to form meta-representations (although he did not suggest a reason for this impairment), thus causing their documented pretend-play deficit. However, during the 1980's and into the 1990s, more and more research began to challenge the meta-representational model as an explanation of autism. For example, Lewis and Boucher in 1988 found that *high-functioning* children with autism (mental ages averaging around that of a 5 year-old) were able to engage in the pretend or symbolic play equal to that of typically developing children. This finding threw the whole concept of meta-representation into question, and the same authors even replicated this research in 1995 (Lewis and Boucher, 1995). What was interesting about this controversial research was that the children with autism did not engage in pretend play *spontaneously or with novelty*; they needed to be cued and pressured to engage in pretend play. More research that followed (e.g., Charman et al. 1997) found similar results, suggesting that something other than a deficit in meta-representational thinking was perhaps at the core of autism. Unfortunately, most of these studies used "high-functioning" participants as noted above, which further complicated what the findings meant, and what could possibly be going on to cause the emergence of autism.

The concept of meta-representations was exciting at the time, because it gave a number of researchers a concept to explain autism that most people could understand. It was relatively simple and intrinsically appealing to a variety of researchers (e.g., Happe 1994; Frith 1989), and it explained a great deal of behavior related to autism. So when research emerged that contradicted these ideas, the challenges were reluctantly acknowledged because some had expanded upon the ideas dramatically. For example, Baron-Cohen (1996) had proposed that meta-representation allowed people to imagine and understand the minds of others. He called this process the development of a "theory of mind" or "ToM." In his book on what came to be known as "mindblindness," Baron-Cohen suggested that typically developing persons develop the ability to imagine or cognitively represent the states of mind of others. This can then be extended to imagining states of mind of the self during insight or self-reflection. Simply put, ToM allowed someone to "think about" the human states of mind. The model for ToM that Baron-Cohen developed became a quite complex and comprehensive four-component system. It began with, interestingly, an "<u>intent</u> detector" and an "<u>eye</u> detector," that combined to create "triadic representations," which culminated in mature ToM. To explain the source of these skills, Baron-Cohen posited they were the outcome of a long, evolutionary process, and then the subsystems leading to ToM simply came "on-board." For persons with autism, something went awry in this progression; it is not clear what, but something went awry. To demonstrate an impaired ToM in persons with autism, Baron-Cohen used the "Sally Anne" task. In research using this technique (where items are moved without certain characters knowing they have been moved), Baron-Cohen et al. (1985) found that most <u>but not all</u> children with autism were unable to correctly assume the mental perspective of the various characters in a story. So like the research in pretend play, certain children with autism were able to perform as a typically developing child would. However, the majority of the children with autism tended to respond in a "non-thinking-about" manner rather than a meta-representational manner.

So, given the variability for persons with autism on the Sally Anne task and variability in pretend play, where does this leave the meta-representational model? If one conceives of meta-representation (or for that matter, imagination as we have defined it) as an "all or none" ability and hence the mechanisms that allow for the creation of imagination need to be either on or off, then we can dismiss the whole idea of meta-representation as being the core of autism because clearly, some children with autism can demonstrate some form of these behaviors some of the time. But what if it was not an "all or none" ability? What if one could develop these abilities to a degree? Is it possible to develop a little imagination? And if so, how would it happen and what would it look like?

Back to Peter Hobson

The work done by Peter Hobson creates an excellent example of the emergence of more and more sophisticated levels of mature thinking, and what this might mean for the child with autism. For Hobson, the very young, typically developing infant is highly attuned to the social behavior of others quite naturally, and he or she is continually watching, gazing, and imitating the immediate behaviors of those around them. Then there is a dramatic shift in thinking at the end of the first year of development and into year two, signifying a real change: the infant is now able to think about objects with the parent in a referential way, gesturing, showing, pointing, and both referencing and taking on the emotional attitude and responses of the parent. Awareness of the other person's intentional and emotional relation to an object comes "online;" or, in other words, the infant can now begin the process of developing the capacity to imagine the thinking and emotions of people, laying groundwork for a host of other skills that rely on this ability such as pretend play, empathy, language, embarrassment, and a concept of self. Not coincidentally, all of these skills, including those seen early in life as well as those that develop later in the typical child, are impaired in autism to some degree. Hobson suggests that the typical infant is 'innately equipped' to perform certain early behaviors and maintain emotional connectedness with the parent, and he provides us with a mechanism or process by which this entire evolution in thinking takes place: identification.

In the next chapter, we will discuss what the concept of identification is, how it is related to the psychoanalytic (Freudian) school of object relations, and why identification has been generally disregarded in the field of autism. It turns out that researchers in the field of autism have a pretty good reason for avoiding identification, but I don't want to get ahead of myself. Hobson (2002), on the other hand, had no problem presenting this concept as central to the development of thinking, and therefore central to autism. Consider this quote:

"More than this: thinking arises out of repeated experiences of moving from one psychological stance to another...The mechanism by which all this occurs is the process of identification...To identify with someone is to assume the other person's stance or characteristics...The critical element in this kind of identifying I am describing is that it involves feelings and attitudes. This kind of identifying does more than change a person's actions – it changes the person's subjective experience of the world." (p.105)

Hobson (2005) further suggests that identification creates the mental space for more complex levels of thinking, and that it is precisely this process that causes the problems seen in persons with autism:

"By means of this process of identification in the context of triadic person-person-world relations, they are lifted out of their one-track, inflexible perspective to apprehend things and events 'according to the other.' This process is not only critically disrupted in children with autism, but also critically important for the development of context-sensitive symbolic thinking." (p. 417)

But we need to be careful in how we are conceiving of this deceptively simple process called "identification." Even in the above passages, it is not entirely clear what is happening. Is the child actively and naturally assuming or taking on the "stance" of another, or is the child being "lifted" out of one-track thinking by some external force? What actually happens in the process of identification? Understanding this concept is important because it is suggested that due to this process of identification, the infant comes to see that the parent perceives the infant; the infant then realizes that she can be the object of another person's perception. What this creates is self-awareness and the ability to perceive the self as an object of evaluation, which leads to embarrassment, shyness, or coy behaviors demonstrated later in development. Simply put, it is the (usually) "automatic" process of identification that allows for the creation of the mental space to think about, which underlies so many other skills yet to be developed in the child. As Hobson (2002) states:

"It is because what is internal becomes external, and what is external may be internalized, that relationships can promote the development of a capacity to think, even in adulthood." (p. 175)

Part 2: Emergence of the Dynamic Behavior Theory of Autism (DBT-A)

Chapter 5: Our Love-Hate Relationship with Psychoanalysis and Identification

It seems like a simple enough word, identification, yet it is really quite a complex concept when one examines its history in psychology, and more specifically within psychoanalysis and the related schools that have emerged from Freudian thinking over the years. We will discuss this in time, but for the moment, think about what the word might mean to the layperson. Identification, as we mentioned above, was used by Hobson to mean the assumption of the "stance" or "characteristics" of another person. But if you use the term in everyday conversation, it often has a wider meaning. You might say to someone, "I can identify with what you are saying," meaning that you can easily imagine the other person's perspective or line of thinking. Or you might say, "Our group is identified as conservative," meaning that your membership unifies you with others in an idea or ideal. Identification has many related terms such as 'identity' or 'identical,' which in their own right, imply a unified sameness or oneness. These terms as a group suggest that identification can mean more than a similarity between two things; it can infer an actual unification, where two entities are actually considered one and the same thing. Or consider this somewhat different definition which is more in line with the form of identification we are interested in:

"A largely unconscious process whereby an individual models thoughts, feelings, and actions after those attributed to an object that has been incorporated as a mental image."   Mirium-Webster, 2007

Interestingly, this definition is from a medical dictionary because identification is subsumed under the psychoanalytic perspective, which is the traditional orientation of psychiatrists. Notice the part on incorporation of a "mental image." A "psychoanalytic" orientation is synonymous with Freudian ideas, but this is actually an area that has evolved over time and taken many twists and turns since the early part of the 20th century. So many twists and turns in fact, that we need to limit our discussion to one of the most recent and significant incarnations of Freudian ideas, the school of "object relations."

Before we move on to this area, you may have noticed from the definition above that we are going to have another problem with terminology in discussing identification within object relations. This time we are not missing a good word as in the case of "thinking about" and "imagination," but rather we have one word with two meanings. The problem comes with the word "object," which most people understand to be something inanimate, like a brick or a spoon. In psychoanalytic circles, the term "object" is used more broadly to mean the aim of a psychological drive, usually the person to or with whom another person is relating. Simply put, in psychoanalytic schools an object is usually a person, and what is of interest is how that person-as-object is identified with and incorporated into another person's psyche. Incorporation can and does create the "mental image" of the person noted above, or more importantly, the internal representation of the relationship with that person-object. As defined by Michael St. Clair (1996), an object is "the 'other' involved in a relationship or, from an instinctual point of view, that from which the instinct gets gratification" (p.219). Nevertheless the object being a person is not an absolute; there is actually no clear requirement in psychoanalytic theory that an object must be a person. In one of the most widely cited texts on the various schools of psychoanalytic thinking, Greenberg and Mitchell (1983) plainly state this. That means that at least from a psychoanalytic standpoint, an object could, in fact, be an inanimate object, or in the more traditionally Freudian use of the term, it could be a person. In fact, in discussing the complex process of identification in detail, Schafer (1968) notes:

"The subject may, of course, identify with representations of nonhuman creatures and things as well as with those of other persons. Identifications with pets, wild animals, and machines, to give a few examples, are not rare." (p. 142)

This is important because as we have seen, the process of identification has been suggested to play a core role in how we develop the ability to think, so knowing how we are identifying may be as important as knowing with what we are identifying.

So what is the role of an "object" within the recent incarnation of Freudian ideas called "object relations"? Note that there have been many changes made to Freud's original ideas over the years, and object relations is just one such interpretation. While most people think that psychoanalysts are mired in Freud's original focus on sexuality and dealing with our naughty ids, Freudian thinking has actually quietly moved on and continues to be the core training mode for psychiatrists and many psychologists. In the school of object relations, early experiences with parents create an important template or lens through which we all understand or see our own world. For better or for worse, the idea is that how we related to our parents and how they responded to us as children "lays the track" as it were, for later functioning with other "objects" or people. As we grow older, those very early relationships are acted out in our adult relations. So, for example, let's say that as a young child, you secretly resented your father's over-bearing and authoritarian 'pushing around' of your mother and other people in your life. As you grow older, when you encounter persons in authority (like a teacher or a boss), your tendency is to re-enact this early "object-relation" with your father, and you (for reasons you don't see or understand) might inappropriately challenge or obstruct this person. Anger would quickly and easily rise to the top in these types of situations, and you would not be able to enjoy a neutral and balanced emotional response. This type of problem would be a common one that someone brings to therapy, asking, "Why do I do this? It is causing so many problems in my life..." Because the answer is hiding in the very way that person was trained early on to see the world, the very obvious answer remains a mystery. That patient's own psychological "tracks" are part and parcel of who they are; so much so that they can't see what is happening. One of the goals of therapy based on object relations ideas is to illuminate these patterns, so the patient can become aware of what he or she is thinking and doing. Once you are aware of where the emotion comes from, you can more easily work through the associated emotions and decide whether or not to change the pattern.

So while most people think that an analyst is going to ask a lot of questions about your past and early childhood (and he or she might be interested in this area), it is actually the novel and new encounter with the therapist that is of central interest. Just like our relationships with others in our world, the patient begins quite naturally to weave the same types of relations with the neutral therapist, re-creating bits and pieces of earlier "relations" with past "objects." Presented with this very unusual relationship, the patient acts in the manner known best to him, creating the stuff of "transference" that the therapist notes and considers. As the patient continues to "transfer" his understanding of the world onto the therapist, the patterns brought forth illuminate the patient's general take on the world, and even his relationship with himself. The very manner in which the patient functions psychologically is exposed through this process, and the skilled psychoanalyst acknowledges it, understands it, and in time, gives it back to the patient in a way that (hopefully) leads to insight, understanding, and subsequent improved functioning on the part of the patient. This is not a simple process; the therapist cannot and should not open a wound he or she cannot help close. And the therapist not only has to manage the patient's thinking and behavior, but his or her response to the patient; this is "counter-transference" that can provide important information about the patterns that are becoming evident. But the core idea is that what is enacted with the therapist represents what the patient felt and experienced as a young child, and being able to put these emotions and thoughts on the table in a safe environment will lead to growth. So this idea that how one experienced the world early on creates how one thinks and feels today, bears some vague resemblance to what we have been discussing up to this point; that early relations with others might create the very manner in which we think. So have psychoanalysts considered this? It turns out they have.

The Ugly Psychoanalytic Past of Autism

One of the reasons that psychoanalytic theory has been at best neglected in research on and treatment for autism has to do with an early psychiatrist, Bruno Bettleheim, who unfairly and incorrectly blamed the emergence of autism on the mother. If you have seen the movie on Temple Grandin, you have seen the tremendous damage that can be done by assuming such as stance. But at the time, we knew very little about autism, and it seemed to be rarely diagnosed. Bettleheim proposed that autism was the result of the mother withholding sufficient affection from her children, resulting in a poor emotional connection. The father was also blamed but to a lesser degree, mainly due to his weak or ineffectual presence in the child's early life. But the blame none-the-less fell squarely on the shoulders of the parents, resulting in the popular term "refrigerator mother." The theory basically suggested that the emotional "coldness" of the mother of the child with autism was at the core of this disorder, and these ideas remained the central explanation for autism for decades. Even though there were typically developing children present in the families of a child with autism and mothers with warm, compassionate, and caring personalities, this theory became popular and the damage done remains a hot-spot topic in autism research and treatment. In fact, while the essence of the observation-based, behavioral model is antithetical to abstract, internal, psychoanalytic approach, this does not capture the intense resistance to and common derogation of psychoanalytic thinking in many autism circles. In my experience, any reference to these ideas is at best met with skepticism and suspicion, but more often with outright rejection and even anger. Mention analytic ideas to a behaviorist and chances are, you will not receive a good response.

While I am not a proponent of Bettleheim's archaic ideas, I am also not ready to throw out the proverbial baby with the bathwater. So let's begin at the beginning and re-focus on the psychoanalytic concept that may help us better understand autism, identification. Freud introduced the idea of identification in the early 1900's (Freud, 1917), and then expanded the ideas in later revisions of his theory. One of the best explanations he gave of identification was in his famous introductory lectures (Freud, 1932), where he described it as a type of assimilation in that one person becomes so like the other person that it was as if one was taking the other "up into itself" (p.63). This would again suggest more of a type of unification or merger, where one person was not only "like" the other person, but temporarily actually is the other person in a manner of speaking. This extends beyond Hobson's conceptualization of identification as the assumption of "characteristics," to include the very being of the other person. Such an idea is hardly news to the psychoanalytic community, as psychoanalysts such as W. R. D. Fairbairn (Fairbairn, 1941) suggested a nearly complete merger with the parent at a very early age, or in psychoanalytic-object terms, a "state of identification with the object." Interestingly, not only have psychoanalysts in the recent past focused on identification, but they have also delved into the 9-month revolution in thinking ideas that we have been discussing, albeit in a characteristically abstract manner.

For example, a renowned psychoanalyst, Edith Jacobson (1964), talked about the role of objects in the development of infantile thinking at exactly the point in development with which we are concerned:

"As the child enters his second year of life, changes in the nature of his relations to the object world set in...they mark the introduction into the psychic organization of a new time category, the concept of future. Moreover, they presuppose the ability to distinguish...differences between objects – animate and inanimate – as well as between objects and the self." (p. 49)

Jacobson's position was that the process of identification (and the object with which the individual identified) typically replaced the state of most primitive self and other fusion, and that the resultant self-image was a function of the internalized traits and parts of the other person or object (Fonagy & Target, 2003). She continues later in the 1964 volume, to discuss how the process of identification also leads to ever-expanding sectors of the developing mind:

"Object and self awareness grows, perception and organization of memory traces expand. The object imagery gradually extends to the animate and inanimate world. Language symbols, functional motor activity, and reality testing develop." (p. 53)

Or consider the following discussion of how symbolic thinking derives from early emotional experiences from Otto Kernberg, one of the best known object relations theorists living today (quoting Otto Kernberg in Sandler, 1987):

"Shifting from consideration of the minimal requirements for the assumption of symbolic thinking to that of the development of a subjective sense of self, I have proposed that this development may be conceived as taking place in at least three stages: (a) an early state of primary consciousness or subjectivity, first activated during peak affect states and characterized solely by affective experiences without any sense of self; (b) a later stage of self-awareness, that is, a reflective awareness of a subjective state that differs from other subjective states, and (c) an integrated sense of self as the basis for a self-reflective awareness of any particular subjective state – the "categorical self" of the philosophers. Self awareness is now not only that of temporally changing subjective experiences while a "self looks on" but a clear awareness of a continuous entity of subjective self as something stable against which each subjective state is evaluated." (p. 97)

For Kernberg, identification results in the self modeling itself on the selected object, which is typically the parent (Fonagy & Target, 2003). Thus psychoanalysts have been thinking about thinking for some time, and creating theories for many years that touch upon how early experiences create the psychological world of the infant.

But because the thrust of psychoanalysis was the goal of an effective form of therapy for adult persons, the role of ideas such as those noted above was often of secondary import; they were of interest (usually) only to the extent that they supported or informed what was happening in the adult mind. If psychoanalysts were interested in what happened in early childhood, it was often only because it helped them understand the roots of later borderline personality disorders, depressions, or psychotic conditions. In fact, direct links between early development and disorders that emerge later in life are common in psychoanalytic literature (e.g., Horner, 1984). Even our central concept of identification was considered commonly (although certainly not exclusively) serving development a bit later than the one- to two-year-old period we are interested in. For example, identification with the mother or father formed basic sexual dispositions as an outcome of the Oedipal process which was considered active during year three to year five. This is not to say that identification was not active during earlier formative years; only that it was a different kind of identification, sometimes called *primary* identification or what Kernberg called "introjection." Remember that in discussing autism, we see problems in developing imaginative functions or "thinking about" that emerge late in the first year of life and then become more apparent into the second year when a clearer diagnosis can be established. Because of this, any discussion of identification needs to be of the most basic sort, that which is evident or hypothesized during year one.

So what is this thing we are calling primary identification? Primary identification is a particularly chaotic and affect-laden state, where the self and object (usually the mother) are considered "non-differentiated." You may be wondering what this means, and simply put, during this stage of identification, the child does not merely assume the "characteristics" or "stance" of the mother, but is in fact, one with the mother. This is considered an early state of unification or "merger" with the mother, where she or another significant caretaker functions as the organizing or holding psychological vessel for the infant. (It is actually the process of secondary identification where the infant takes into the self-representation the more commonly considered characteristics or attributes of the object (Sandler 1987).) It is primary identification that results in the creation of the infant's framework for the genesis of his or her subjective world; the infant's formation of their own self-representation via the "taking in" of the maternal "object." The famous psychoanalyst Margaret Mahler (Mahler et al., 1975) suggested a similar form of identification when she proposed that the very young infant became "symbiotic" with the mother, or quite naturally entered into an undifferentiated physical and psychological state with the mother. The symbiotic "dual unity" of mother and child laid the very foundations of healthy thinking and personality functions:

"Within the symbiotic common orbit, the two partners or poles of the dyad may be regarded as polarizing the organizational and structuring processes. The structures that derive from this double frame of reference represent a framework to which all experiences have to be related before there are clear and whole representations in the ego of the self and the object world (Jacobson, 1964). Spitz (1965) calls the mother the auxiliary ego of the infant. Similarly, we believe the mothering partner's "holding behavior"…is the symbiotic organizer – the midwife of individuation, of psychological birth." (p. 47)

Successful unification and attachment with the mother preceded later "hatching" or psychological separation in the second year of development, from what Mahler called the "symbiotic orbit" of mother and child. Healthy and successful navigation of this process resulted in strong psychic structures that came to represent what was "self" and what was not self. In other words, identification is much more than one entity deciding to being similar to, take on characteristics of, or be "like" another entity; from a psychoanalytic standpoint, primary identification means, at least for a while, child and parent are psychologically one dual unit. And while they are one, parts of the basic roadmap of how to think are transferred from the parent as object, to the child.

This is an important idea because it means that the type of identification we are interested in involves the child more or less *becoming* the mother or "object" with whom (or with which) the child identifies. In other words, the child becomes able to think as a result of the early, successful identification process, and so the process of identification becomes as important as the actual object selected. Before we move on, it is important to touch on one other aspect of primary identification with the maternal "object." In psychoanalysis, the taking in of an object is often thought of as progressive; sometimes from a "part-object" state to a "whole-object" state. This is easily understood when applied to later development, when only certain aspects of objects are perceived. For example, a young person or adult may be able to only see positive or only negative aspects of that other person. As you might expect, this creates problems because they are not "seeing" the "whole" person or object as it really is, just the parts they can tolerate or comprehend. Sometimes this is referred to as only being able to see the world and the people in it in "black and white," rather than being able to accept that people are mostly "grays." By this I mean that people are almost always combinations and degrees of opposing traits; they are good and bad, cooperative and obstructive, loving and unkind. In psychoanalysis, a mark of successful and well-functioning development is being able to see people in the world as "grays," whereas seeing only certain aspects of people is a defensive function designed to keep out ambivalence that might overwhelm a fragile psychological system. This defensive function is sometimes referred to as "splitting," although this term has other meanings and applications as well.

But we are interested in a much earlier and much more primitive application of this concept. This line of psychodynamic theory suggests that even very early development typically proceeds from part- to whole-object understanding. In the stage of development that we are interested in, namely primary identification where the infant temporarily is the parent psychologically, the part-object for the developing infant might be a bottle or human body part, such as a breast or hand. This understanding moves on to a "whole object" orientation, where, for example, there is a more complete or more inclusive and whole father or mother object. This perceived whole-object would have a range of human properties as noted by Fairbairn (1954). Another psychoanalyst, Schafer (1968), talked about this part to whole process further when he wrote:

"Psychological development includes increasing ascendency of the secondary process: object representations…tend toward complex differentiations…they tend toward objective wholeness in the sense of encompassing and organizing enough significant physical and psychological attributes of an object to constitute a substantial, specific, and enduring human figure…" (p. 144)

So what happens if you consider the idea of part- to whole-object understanding during the very early stage of primary identification? We already know that the very young infant "is" what they identify with, which may or may not be a whole human object. In the chapters that follow, I will suggest an alternative theoretical explanation derived from these ideas that better integrates what we have learned about the symptoms of autism, how thinking develops, and more discrete behaviors and skills such as pretend play and symbolic thinking.

As we discussed previously, research has not fully supported the representational/meta-representational model of autism. The present psychoanalytic approach might better explain what we know about autism by expanding upon Hobson's concept of identification. Specifically, as I have stated previously (Woodard & Van Reet, 2011):

"Primary identification is a process by which the very mind of the infant is constructed by the object, nonliving or living, with which he or she identifies. The "stuff" of identifications is derived from the perceived world of the infant, or the objects that are in fact nonliving things and people. Note, however, that even people are, from an analytic orientation, perceived first in part-object form; it is only with transitional time and integration of the person as a whole-object that understanding evolves from a collection of things or parts to a living being that has the capacity to imagine. We propose that the distinction between an inanimate object and a whole human object is central to how the typically developing mind is structured and created, given these voluntary imaginative functions or abilities of the whole human object." (p. 220)

Allow me to state it another way. The developing
infant psychologically becomes that with which he or
she identifies. If the developing infant does not, as
most infants quite naturally and easily do, navigate
completely from a part-object to a whole-object
orientation, they will hence perceive the world and the
self in the manner reflective of the degree of this
progression. That is, if I identify with a part-object
which would be an inanimate object or non-whole or
non-human object, <u>so will my thinking be</u>. And while it
seems to go without saying, inanimate objects as you
know, can't imagine or "think about," can they?

Chapter 6: What It Means to Identify with an Object

We have now discussed many of the essentials that are necessary for proposing a new theory of autism based on the concept of identification. We have discussed the main and associated symptoms, and enough about genetics and treatment to leave us a bit perplexed as to what autism is, where it comes from, and how it evolves. We know that there is simply no single gene that leads to the expression of autism (yet there are certainly genetic forces at play), and behavioral treatments have only moderate effects mainly because the etiology is so poorly understood. However, the timing and nature of the disorder has led us to focus on the 9-month revolution in thinking, which is a period in development suspected to be of central importance by a number of researchers in the area of autism. But how is this early process related to autism? What actually happens to cause this disorder? Is there some semblance of ideas or concepts that you and I can use to at least get a basic understanding of what is happening? The theories that seek to explain the 9-month revolution in thinking are complicated not only by their abstract form (thinking about thinking is not easy), but also by the challenges of infant development research and the fact that so many different things are taking place at the same time as a child grows. But as a group, in the thinking realm, they suggest that what we consider normal human thinking is derived from a certain type of pervasive, early relationship with the world; specifically, early relationships with people in the world. Because these types of concepts are far beyond the reaches of the predominant behavioral perspective, we need to venture into areas traditionally "off-limits" to researchers in autism.

While undoubtedly unpopular, we need to draw upon a perspective where the currency is not what is seen and measured, but rather what is abstract, non-observable, and purely psychological conceptualization, supported only by what we think the infant is thinking.

Because the area of autism is dominated by behaviorally-oriented professionals, this might be a hard pill to swallow. But if we are to move forward, even if some might feel this is a step backward, we need to expand our exploration into areas that may very well have something to offer alongside a well-conducted functional behavior analysis. The area of purely psychological conceptualization that deals in the period of development we are interested in is the psychoanalytic concept of identification. We have discussed how we are less interested in the more common secondary type of identification, and more focused on primary identification. It is during primary identification that the parent and child unify, and create the bond or relationship that some developmental theorists believe is so unnamable that only a poet or painter could actually capture what is happening at this time. It is this period of primary identification that I am suggesting is central to the emergence of autism not only due to the timing of this type of identification in relation to when we see autism first emerge, but also because it is during primary identification that certain aspects of the early templates of thinking are hypothesized to be forged and provided to the infant via symbiotic joining with the parent. That is to say that the choice of the object identified with and the extent to which whole objects are integrated into thinking over part-objects, makes an important and unique contribution to the overall process of core, "thinking-about" cognitive development. This is first evident in the infant, and then can continue to affect thinking and behavior as the person continues to mature across the lifespan.

Let me try to be as clear as possible: to make further progress in understanding autism and related treatment, or at least to create a theory that can suggest testable hypotheses, we must meld behavioral, developmental, <u>and</u> psychoanalytic thinking. We can draw upon the major contribution of the psychoanalytic school to the extent to which psychoanalysts have conceived of, as Margaret Mahler puts it, the psychological birth of the human infant. More specifically, I am suggesting that:

For a variety of reasons, the infant on the trajectory for autism comes into the world with a propensity or preference for inanimate objects and part-object identification as compared to human object and whole-object identification. These are not mutually exclusive states, but better conceived as a continuum of identification options. Primary identification contributes to the emerging cognitive structure by influencing interactive components: 1) how we understand, conceive of, and perceive of the world around us, and 2) the level of complexity or sophistication in how we think "about," which is derived from the extent to which a whole human object is chosen. These factors affect not only thinking and associated behaviors in infancy and across the lifespan, but also how we conceive of abstract concepts such as the self. Thus, the spectrum of autism disorders are, for all intents and purposes, outcomes of variations in or insults to the early thinking "about"/imaginative capacity. The infant's propensity for the inanimate and part-object end of the continuum may be sufficient for autism to emerge, or may be further propelled by environmental factors. This means that 1) influencing elements would be any genetic or environmental factor that influences or contributes to placement or movement on the hypothesized continuum, and 2) treatment would be effective only to the extent that placement or movement towards the human/whole object end of the continuum is achieved.

That being said, we can proceed by first delineating what this supposed continuum might look like as a stand-alone concept, and then as it relates to autism. Next, we will look at supporting evidence as to why this might be a reasonable way to conceive of autism (which is extensive). And finally, we will discuss one element that is hypothesized as contributing to the increased prevalence of autism: our continually emerging and increasing cultural obsession with objects.

In my 2011 article (Woodard & Van Reet, 2011), we discussed the continuum that I have here again proposed, but perhaps now we can expand on it more fully. We suggested that the inanimate to human object concepts needed to be considered in concert with the idea of part to whole psychological development. These awkward terms are, at present, the best we have to convey the main thrust of this area, and are complicated by the fact that even people are, at first, perceived in part-object form. It is only with time that a person potentially comes to be understood by the infant as a whole person or unit. But what do we mean by a "whole" person? How can we better understand what leads up to this typical and normal state of identification? I have suggested that it might makemore sense to begin in this uncharted theoretical territory with four main demarcations of identification as follows (with acronyms slightly altered from the original):

1) Part-object/Inanimate object (PI) Identification (Least sophisticated)
2) Part-object/Emerging Human (EH) Identification
3) Incomplete Whole Human (IH) Identification
4) Whole Human (WH) Identification (Most sophisticated)

We will discuss each of these possible forms of identification on the continuum in turn, first from a general theoretical standpoint, and then in terms of how each might further explain what is seen in autism. This discussion builds upon what was outlined in the 2011 article.

The first form of identification (PI) suggests that the infant, for any number of possible reasons, has oriented toward part-objects and inanimate objects, and away from human objects, for identification. Interestingly, a similar observation was made by Margaret Mahler more than thirty years ago, but never fully developed. Mahler (1979a) notes that, in what she calls autistic infantile psychosis, the mother "remains a part object, seemingly devoid of specific cathexis and *not distinguished from inanimate objects*" (italics added) (p. 135). She continues, "This autistic psychotic child was characterized (as were all those whom I observed) by a peculiar inability to discriminate between living and inanimate objects, even in a perceptual sense" (p. 138). Mahler (1979b) even provides an example of non-human identification during the symbiotic phase in her case presentation of Harriet, and the mechanical outcomes:

"As early as at eight months, she consoled herself and enjoyed nothing more than rocking back and forth before a large mirror in an autoerotic fashion, watching herself and thus reinforcing the kinesthetic sensations... Her preference for inanimate objects over people was striking. Her identifications were with dolls, or at best, with the family dog... The not-yet fourteen-month- old little girl seemed to oblige mechanically." (p. 115)

Given what we know about identification, what could we hypothesize identification with an object might further look like? Most obviously, there would be an interest in things as much as people, although if an aversion to the sound or presence of people was present, inanimate objects would likely be preferred over people. To the observer though, even an equal level of interest in things and people would likely appear to be, as compared to typical development, an unusual disinterest in people. Further, it would be sensible to assume that certain things could be attached to and appear nearly obsessional in their importance; much as a typically developing infant clings to the mother, an infant with a PI level of identification would cling to things. With respect to the idea of the identification object creating the manner in which we see the world, every object in the world (including people) would necessarily only have inanimate object status. In other words, things would be things and people would be things, because the uniquely human thinking properties had not developed in the early identification process. The infant who remains at the PI level of identification could and would perceive the world (both objects and people) in the most basic inanimate object form, and the capacity for understanding the unique qualities of living things, such as volitional thought and emotion, would not emerge. Given this, both things and people would be <u>treated</u> as if they were things; both my relation with things and my relationships with people would be emotion-less and mechanical.

It does not take much imagining to think of what this might look like for the infant progressing through the end of the first year of life and into year two: equal interest in or a preference for inanimate objects over people, the treatment of people as if they were objects, the treatment of other living objects as things – say, the family dog, and an absence of interest in the indicators of thinking and emotion in others, namely joint attention and social referencing. As a side note, I am unclear on how this course of events would affect object permanence. At first I suggested that because it is an imagination-based skill (which is dependent on human identification), a PI level of identification would bar its emergence, but it is also a skill that uniquely emerges prior to the 9-month revolution in thinking. This may suggest that it is a skill somehow unique in psychological, thinking development. Perhaps research in this area would clarify the role of object permanence, exploring: is there a difference between object permanence skills in the most severely autistic children (those with no spoken language, absent reciprocal socialization, and repetitive behavior) as compared to those less severely affected? An answer of "yes," which I suspect would be the case, would suggest that the identification process is having the expected effect this skill area. However, a "no" would support its unique properties, perhaps related to the pure object qualities and developmental timing of this particular skill area.

Returning to the idea of everything in the environment as having only "thing" status, to imagine this, we could conceive of all living things as machines or robots. Note that we need to use the real kind of robots in this exercise, not the emotion-laden and entertaining ones often represented in movies. All the living things in our world would move and do this or that, but without any emotion or voluntary original thought. If you or I came in contact with one of these "machines," we would likely treat it as such; we might touch it or turn it, or use it as it is designed to meet our immediate needs, but that is all we would do because we understand it to be a thing. Or, we might ignore it if it bears no particular use for us at this time. You can't insult a machine, so we would simply go on our way. To you or me, this thing might be of interest because it does move and can do something it is designed to do, but beyond that, it is simply an object in our environment with some features of interest that many of the other objects do not possess. On the other hand, imagine adding to this exercise what you and I know to be true; these "robots" are not machines, but rather living beings with original thinking and emotion. Because of this, the person at the PI level of identification would perceive these particular "robots" as inconsistent and at times, unpredictable machines. They would, by their very nature, violate many of the rules of things by behaving differently for any number of reasons (e.g., a new thought on how to do something, an attempt to substitute one thing for another, the result of a change in emotional state, etc.). It seems that this might make people a bit aversive to the person perceiving people in the world in this manner; how long would you want to keep around your unpredictable robot?

When I say "the rules of things" I am referring to the physical rules that one would expect the child at the PI level of identification to use to conceive of the world. Things typically do not move on their own, change form or shape, come or go on their own, or use original thought or emotion to guide their behavior; that's what makes them things. Once typically developing infants see behavior that indicates this particular type of thinking and emotion— the kind that humanized, emotional robots have, they would become fascinated with the prospect of a thing crossing over to having uniquely human thinking. This is the stuff of many a good sci-fi story. But at the PI level, we would conceive of an expectation of constancy, for everything from my lamp today being a lamp tomorrow, to having things in a certain formation. But we need to be careful not to move into the next level of identification which allows the person with autism to base rules of constancy on how things "should" be; this denotes a primitive ability to think "about" which is not present in this most basic PI level. So constancy for this level of identification would need to be limited to how one knows the world to be based on memory and experience, rather than a more categorizational, comparative, or conceptual knowledge of how it "should" be. Memory after all, is not necessarily affected by the identification process, but rather limited by the level of thinking sophistication that results from the identification process. In other words, much like associative learning remaining basically intact but limited, memory would continue to function within the confines of an absence of the ability to think "about." It would be more of what we think of a "recognition" memory, and less of what would be "recall" memory; the person would know something when they saw it, but pulling the idea up in one's mind and reconstructing it or altering it from the original would not be possible. This idea may become clearer as we continue our discussion on what a PI level of identification means to the process of thinking and the emerging concept of self.

For the person at the PI level of identification, one would expect that changes from or alterations to the original of any number of things might be alarming, but we can also conceive of how they might be fascinating. For you and I to conceive of some version of this, imagine both our amusement and our dismay when we watch a magician do things that we know to be physically impossible. The more rule-violating the trick is, the better the act. But now remove from the equation your knowledge that it is only a trick performed by someone whose job is to create illusion. Suddenly the experience becomes both amazing and a bit unsettling, if not downright terrifying. Much like the robot that has become unpredictable, violations of the rules of the physical environment has the potential to confuse, worry, and alarm us. At the PI level of identification, this response is not because we are afraid of what "could" happen as a result (that would again require thinking "about"), but because what we know to be one way is suddenly different; it is "incorrect." It does not take much imagining to conceive of the continual state of stress that might quickly ensue with a PI level of identification. I would suggest that this concept is one source of the high stress we see in persons with autism as they develop.

In addition to 1) things and people being of equal importance, 2) people being conceived of as things and treated as such, and 3) a preference for constancy, I would expect that the PI level of identification would be marked by a fascination with parts of things rather than the whole. Our theory suggests that an object orientation is associated with "part" versus "whole" conceptualization, which would lead one to expect that individual parts of things (which include people at this level) might bear special interest. Objects as things in what you and I consider to be whole form would not be perceived by the person at a PI level of identification. Rather, they would have an interest in sections, portions, or parts of things, and we would expect them to seek these parts out: a hand would not be part of a whole person, a button would not be part of a larger toy, and a doorknob would not be part of a door. These would all be individual parts, each bearing their own level of importance or significance. Because of this, they would be treated as such; there would be, for example, an interest in what you or I consider to be unusual details of a thing or a part that typically one would ignore or perceive only as serving a subordinate function to the entirety of the object. Interestingly, if we begin to combine aspects of what we would expect a person with a PI level of identification to be, we can start to picture how this person might behave. Pairing constancy with a focus on the parts of things, for example, would suggest this person might tend to engage with sections of toys that do the same thing over and over. For example, this person might spin a tire on a toy car continually, rather than use the car as an integrated whole.

Beyond these four likely and more obvious outcomes of primary identification with an object instead of a person, we need to consider how such identification might affect two additional, inseparable concepts: the level of sophistication of thinking and the concept of self. I have suggested that the type and nature of the object chosen for early identification affects not only how we perceive the world as noted above, but also the level of complexity or sophistication of thinking. This is a broad statement given the many functions and skills that we consider to be "thinking," but our theory is made a bit simpler by being able to delineate what makes people so different than most other objects in the world: people think "about" or "imagine" as we have defined and discussed it previously, and have emotions linked to this ability. Many aspects of thinking are, as evidenced by behavior, well underway even at birth and shortly thereafter (e.g., recognition memory, the capacity for associative learning, habituation, and even a basic understanding of the physical rules of the environment), and would not be inhibited necessarily by inanimate object identification. However, the unique contribution that can be made by person-as-object (that is, the ability to think "about" and the experience and understanding of associated emotions (associated because they too must be imagined)), would not be available to the person at the PI level of identification. Such a situation, as one might imagine, could have devastating central effects on the person experiencing this trajectory, and a multitude of secondary effects. Keeping this fairly abstract idea in mind, we can hypothesize how a PI level of identification would affect certain aspects of the person's cognition.

Beginning with early development, the ability to think without the commonly associated ability to think "about" would further propel the infant's disinterest in joint attention and social referencing. This is because the capacity for conceiving of another person's thinking, purpose, or intent would be absent. Similarly, there would be no purpose in following the eye-gaze of another person or pointing out something of interest because other people are not perceived through the capacity to think "about." There would be no social smile or shared enjoyment with another, because the infant at the PI level does not have the capacity to imagine the enjoyment or emotion that the other person is experiencing. Facial expression of others would be inconsequential, because the emotions of others can't be imagined. More specifically, for the infant at the PI level, emotions derived from relationships with other people would be absent. This is not to say that the person at this level would not have emotions anymore than they would not have the ability to think; they would simply be emoted in response to events related to things rather than people, or purely organic experiences such as internally-derived mood. As the infant began to develop further, the absence of the ability to think "about" would necessarily bar the emergence of functional play following stereotypical use of objects, and pretend play would be absent because this behavior is acutely dependent on the ability to imagine. Further, any cognitive function based on symbolization would be out of reach, as these types of abilities require the ability to have one thing "stand for" or represent another. Without this ability, the infant at the PI level would not respond to their name, and spoken language altogether would be tremendously challenging if not altogether impossible. However, because associative learning remains intact, a person at the PI level may appear to understand some language to the extent that certain verbal expressions of others have led to positive reinforcement or punishment consequences that could be drawn from available memory. The more sophisticated emotions of the young child that are dependent on thinking "about" relationships with other people would not emerge: completely absent would be empathy, shyness, guilt, coyness, or embarrassment.

Beyond these early manifestations of the absence of the ability to think "about," later emerging, dependent, and related cognitive capacities would be affected. Time, for example, would remain a complete mystery to the person at the PI level, because the past and the future as concepts must be imagined. Interestingly, this is not to say that there would not be recognition of things and people from the past. But the experience of existence for the person at the PI level would be, by necessity, an ever-present "now." For this reason, concepts such as waiting or linking current behavior with much delayed, future consequences would be difficult. What "could" happen, which is dependent on both the concept of future and the ability to imagine a variety of outcomes, could not be comprehended. For this reason, hypothesizing, problem-solving, or "looking forward to" would be absent. On the other hand, also absent would be worry about future events and fears of what "could" happen; this might initially sound comforting, but one can also imagine the stress of not being able to hypothesize what is likely to happen "next." Further, because it cannot be imagined or integrated as a whole concept, the idea of a physical or psychological "self" would not be possible. The bodily self would simply be a curious set of physical things that are continually nearby, completely disconnected from the absent whole concept of there being a "me." Imagine what a sensory experience would be under these circumstances-- a surprising sensation being experienced but coming from nowhere and being a part of nothing. My leg would not be "my" leg, because there is no me. As a result, what happens to it is likely to be of little consequence, perhaps only until pain is registered, if pain is registered in this situation.

Likewise, the concept of the psychological self as you and I experience it, would be absent for the person at the PI level. This would be true for a number of reasons. First, the concept of "self" is an imagined concept that we build by integrating parts; these are two functions that we already know are incapacitated at the PI level. Second, the early creation of a concept of self is thought to be the result of a culmination of the early thinking "about" skills: the infant not only imagines another person thinking "about" and feeling "about" other things, but the other person is also thinking about and feeling about me. Therefore, there must be a "me." The ability to conceive of a psychological "self" or concept of "me" is clearly acutely dependent on and derived from the early ability to imagine the thinking and feeling of others, and so it is not something that the person at the PI level would be able to create. Much like the curious notion of recognition memory existing but absent a concept of past, or having emotions but not those derived from relationships with others, the concept of self would be consciousness without the thinking-about-dependent elements that you and I are so accustomed to having alongside consciousness: self-awareness, self-concept, and the ability to self-reflect. In other words, the person at the PI level would "be," but would not perceive the self as an existing entity that can be thought "about." But how would we know that a person was functioning in this manner? In addition to the markers discussed so far, I would suggest that, for example, the person at the PI level of identification would have virtually no ability to comprehend death; there would need to be a "me" for there to be the possibility of no "me." It would also be extremely challenging if not impossible for this person to describe himself or herself as a self, or communicate in a way that indicates what he or she is "like," or how he or she tends to "feel" from day to day or moment to moment.

We have discussed a series of indications or expectations based on a PI level of identification: people are perceived as things, on equal par as things, and treated as things without thought or emotion; there is likely a preference for constancy; parts are more interesting than wholes; and cognitive development is impaired wherever thinking "about" is needed. There is little doubt that this set of expectations is beginning to sound a bit familiar to the reader; but there are three additional levels of identification postulated. What happens when there is some movement along the hypothesized continuum?

Chapter 7: Movement Up the Continuum

The PI level of identification is hypothesized to be the most "object" and the most "part" end of the continuum postulated; a nearly complete absence of identification with a human object, an absence of the perception of the whole human object, and an absence of the initial emergence of the ability to think "about" which is typically derived from the human object's unique, same ability. This ability to think "about" or to remind the reader, intersubjectivity-- a second layer of thinking, dual-processing capabilities, or meta-representation-- is barred at the PI level as a result of early inanimate object unification and identification, rather than identification with a human. Without psychological unification with a whole human object that has thinking "about" capabilities, we would not see the linked behaviors that typically emerge during what is known as the 9-month revolution. Recall though that beyond this most absolute level, we have three more main demarcations: Part-object/Emerging Human (EH) Identification, Incomplete Whole Human (IH) Identification, and Whole Human (WH) Identification. What might these look like? The next level of identification, the EH level, suggests that inanimate object identification was not absolute, and that some early placement on or movement on the hypothesized continuum took place. At this level, the infant and child would have a less absolute part-object orientation, and due to partial identification with a human object, he or she would be able to think "about" to a corresponding degree. The many areas touched by the ability to think "about" would be less severely affected, and a wide variation of abilities could emerge as a result.

To better understand what this might look like, we can follow the same descriptive path created in the previous chapter. Note that with a more complete discussion of the PI level, my discussion of the EH level has evolved somewhat from the 2011 text. Theoretically as a result of partial human identification, there would be a somewhat increased interest in other people, perhaps as a special type of thing or a thing with special qualities of movement, a giver of reinforcement, or a most basic understanding of intent. But interactions would retain, to a great degree, the mechanical quality of the PI level. Primitive thinking "about" abilities might allow for basic emotional bonds to certain, select others which would be most apparent when this person was in their presence, but not as apparent when not in their presence. Early separation from a caregiver would likely only be of concern for a very short period, if at all. There would likely remain a preference for constancy and repetition, but we may begin to see early evidence of the ability to adjust to alterations with lessening distress. There would be a lessened focus on parts, or perhaps a beginning integration of wholes, meaning select understanding of how things go together or work together. The EH level would suggest that the developing infant would show minimal joint attention and social referencing, but continue to rely mainly on recognition memory skills. Emotionally there might be emerging or select instances of shared enjoyment, and sporadic interest in the facial expressions of others. Note that in all these areas, there would be the possibility of significant variation, but this theory would suggest that such skills and behaviors would emerge in concert with each other.

The ability to think "about" to a degree would have significant effects on the developing young child in that very primitive and impaired dual-processing becomes possible. While again, there would be significant room for variation, the young child at the EH level should begin to evidence primitive or sporadic functional play as compared to solely stereotypical play. There may be some ability to engage in basic or rehearsed pretend play, but the quality would be poor and engagement would likely remain limited, non-spontaneous, and stilted. Most significant at the EH level of identification would be the potential for basic language, but this also would vary greatly in terms of quantity and quality. Language might be, as with pretend play, awkward, rehearsed-sounding, or otherwise unusual. Because there are only basic thinking "about" abilities at the EH level, language related to <u>physical</u> qualities of the environment should be more easily grasped than more abstract, <u>other-person-based</u> qualities, such as emotion or <u>my</u> (speaking as the other person) likes or dislikes. Because there would remain an unrealized concept of self-as-object derived from more advanced comprehension of the thinking of others, language would likely be marked by an absence of or confusion regarding pronoun usage. "I" or "me" or "you" would have virtually no meaning in the world of the person at the EH level of identification. Similarly, emotions would likely remain a general mystery to the person at the EH level, due not only to the need for intact thinking "about" capacities but also the other-based nature of emotions. Those emotions generated by or derived from relationships with others -- shyness, empathy, guilt, or embarrassment for example, would remain out of reach for the person at the EH level.

Only the most primitive comprehension of emotions (happy, mad, sad, etc.) may be possible.

As the child became a bit older, the availability of partial thinking "about" capacities would allow for minimal comprehension of concepts such as time. For example, the person at this level of identification may be more able to understand "waiting," but more complex versions of time such as, "We will be doing that in three days," or, "You need to wait until 4:00," would remain a frustrating and complex conundrum. At the EH level, we might see problem-solving abilities in the most basic form, and select instances of fear. There would be a primitive comprehension of the body as a more unified thing or object, and disconnectedness of body parts as unrelated units would diminish. However, the more advanced, other-derived concepts of self-awareness or self-reflection would remain absent. The body may be a more unified, physical object, but it could not as yet be thought of in an objectified manner, or the object of another person's thinking. Therefore, the full concept of "self" would remain elusive for the person at the EH level. One other interesting and generally uniquely human quality that might relate to the level of identification would be the presence of humor. Considering the PI level of identification in comparison to the EH level, we would imagine that the person at the PI level might laugh mainly in response to sensory stimulation or internal states. Any humor related to dual meanings ("I was wondering why the baseball got bigger and bigger, and then it hit me") or even when things are different from how they should be (such as wearing a funny hat), would be lost on the person at the PI level. With a person at the EH level, we would expect much the same although there would be the possibility that a rudimentary understanding of physical object or "slapstick" humor may emerge.

At the third hypothesized level of identification, the Incomplete Whole Human (IH) Identification level, expanded human and whole understanding is accomplished. This level of identification would allow the developing infant an improved yet incomplete capacity to think "about" or imagine, and better integration and understanding of wholes versus parts. How might this level of identification manifest? With these improved abilities and capacities, other people could now be perceived as having some concrete thinking capacities, although the more abstract and complex human emotional functions would be more challenging to comprehend and work with. There might be a better understanding of the more basic emotional states in others and the self, but subtle or complex emotions would still be difficult. There would be a clear and preferred understanding of inanimate objects, and while there might be a remaining preference for constancy and repetition, there would also be an improved capacity for flexibility and accommodation to alterations or changes. The person at the IH level would likely want to indulge their thinking and preference for objects, and focus on inanimate object interactions despite an improved awareness and understanding of people as able to think and feel. Related to this idea, some researchers have suggested that high-functioning persons with autism have been able to use parts of the brain typically devoted to object processing for face recognition, instead of using the facial cortex (Scherf et al., 2010). The infant at the IH level would have joint attention with others, but prefer a focus on objects versus people. Some notable social referencing and eye-gaze following however, should be present. There should be improved shared enjoyment, although it too might derive from objects. Some emerging coyness and shyness, as well as stranger anxiety could be present at this level of identification.

A young child at the IH level would have the capacity to engage in functional play, and would understand how parts come together to form a whole to a great degree. This would likely be apparent for object wholeness as compared to people, meaning a complete and deepened understanding of people would remain elusive. Pretend play should be present but not fully consistent with typical play behavior; inanimate objects and ritualized or repetitive play might be preferred over representations of people and play that considers or elaborates on social relation or emotion. Solitary pretend play may be preferred, and others would not likely be drawn into this play activity. Verbal capacities and language would be largely intact, although again, given the preference for objects and constancy, language might be marked by an object or topic focus and rigidity or repetition. Memory functions would have the capacity to develop some abilities to recall in addition to recognition, and problem-solving and hypothesizing would be more possible; they would better happen with inanimate objects as the main topic however, in comparison to people-based challenges. With thinking "about" in place to a greater degree, past and present would become available yet likely be still impaired concepts, and the person at the IH level would begin to be able to fear what "might" happen, especially as it relates to their physical existence. Similarly, the self could be partially conceptualized, but would remain mainly relative to physical object form or facts about the self, with the more abstract emotional qualities being curious, confusing, or simply a mystery. There would likely be limited and primitive self-awareness and perhaps the ability for limited self-reflection if pressured, with special challenges when it comes to one's own emotions. And embarrassment or the constant monitoring of other people's evaluation of one's own behavior, a common aspect of the typically developing child, would likely remain absent. We can quickly imagine the particularly frustrating, confusing, and even painful social existence of the person at the IH level of identification, although with intensive support, approximations of improved social behavior would become possible and have been shown to emerge (Lopata et al., 2010).

Whole human (WH) identification would be associated with the typically developing person, and represented in what is known to be normal (meaning most common) progression in the areas discussed above. The infant would display the full thinking "about," imaginative capacities, and would understand objects and people in whole form. This means that people would become understood both as things existing in space and time in the physical world, as well as distinctly different from objects because they can think and feel. There would be an interest in objects, but a preference for people interactions and all the emotional indicators that this involves. Interactions with others would be marked by fascination and joy, and joint attention, social referencing, eye-gaze following, and shared enjoyment would emerge virtually effortlessly. There would be openness to spontaneity and change, the emergence of functional play and pretend play that integrates things and people, facts and feelings. Others would be drawn into this active play, and preferred over solitary play. There would be the capacity for fully symbolic thinking, normal language development, and the typical emergence of shyness, empathy, stranger anxiety, and embarrassment. The self would be, with time, understood as a whole being, as both a physical object and a thinking and feeling object, and there would be a natural sharing of these unique attributes with the people in their world. The capacity for understanding complex emotions in the self and others would emerge with time, as would the capacity to self-reflect and self-examine. And the continual monitoring of another person's cognitive and emotional response to one's behavior would be present as it is in typically developing persons.

In effect, the WH level of identification would allow to emerge what we understand to be typical thinking-about capacities. By using the ideas of co-occurring inanimate object to human primary identification alongside a part- to whole-object progression, and placing these concepts together on a continuum, one can hypothesize early effects on infant development. As we move along the continuum, the shifting interest in (or focus on) objects and then people, the decreasing insistence on and then preference for physical object constancy, and the evolving part- to whole-object (meaning both inanimate and human objects here) understanding is fairly easily conceived. A bit more challenging is imagining how these shifts or changes in the developmental trajectory would interact with the associated degrees of emergence of the ability to think "about," and how these combinations of events might affect cognition and be demonstrated from a behavioral standpoint. By having worked in the field of developmental disability and autism for nearly two decades, I understand that in describing this continuum and progression I may be influenced by knowing the "end of the story;" but I don't think that this minimizes the tremendous similarities between what may happen at the proposed levels of identification and what we know as the spectrum of autism disorders. In fact, it is the degree of progression on such a continuum that allows us to, for the first time, advance a theory that can accommodate the wide variation of clinical presentations seen in the person with autism. Note also the discipline that this theory could instill in research on autism. Before using research findings to conclude what is or is not representative of autism, this theory would require identification of the severity of the participant group's disorder.   Has the researcher used a group that is best identified by a PI, EH, or IH level of identification and functioning? Vastly different findings would be expected based on this information. Even more confusing would be a "mixed" grouping which would likely lead to an uneven or non-uniform group response to interventions, which is a finding (as we shall see in the next chapter) that is not lost on autism researchers. While identification of cognitive functioning is somewhat helpful, the closest researchers typically come to addressing this issue is the occasional reference to the group being low or high functioning.   The lack of a theoretical framework that is linked to and suggests a logical degree of impairment creates a significant blind-spot at one of the earliest steps in the research process.

The effect that an infant's placement on the proposed continuum has on the behaviors that are representative of the 9-month revolution in thinking, and therefore the emergence of autism, are rather apparent from our discussion. How other-human-based behaviors such as following eye-gaze, eliciting attention of others or joint attention, shared enjoyment, pointing, and showing behavior would be absent or diminished, as well as a preoccupation with parts rather than wholes, and a desire for constancy, repetition, and ritual are all easily derived from this theory. Even empathy being absent, pronoun reversals, the non-existent or incomplete concept of self, impaired pretend play, and absent, unusual, or otherwise impaired language development begin to have a logical source. But what about the other, associated behaviors we mentioned in earlier chapters? Given our newly conceptualized theory, are these behaviors easily understood and explained, or would doing so be more of a "stretch"? Take for example, the tendency for children with autism to use others in a mechanical fashion, as tools in play, and using parts of other people's bodies in unusual ways. A common way that this tendency is evidenced is by the young child with autism placing another person's hand on an object in a manner that does not indicate that the child is touching another human being. Rather, the behavior resembles someone using a set of automated tongs in an effort to get the object to grasp or move another object. Since our theory suggests that people are, to a great extent, conceived of as inanimate objects, this type of behavior is actually quite sensible from such a perspective. Recall our robot example. If your robot was having trouble grasping something, what would you do? You would take its "graspers" (whatever that might be) and help the robot along.

Similarly, we commonly see impairment in gestures for the child with autism. Gestures such as clapping, shaking a finger, or shrugging, are symbolic forms of communication learned only by attending to another person; infants are unlikely to come into the world equipped to shrug. Lacking an interest in the behavior of other people and an inability to think "about" (by letting a body movement represent a communicative meaning), gestures would likely not develop. On the other hand, with time, an older child at the PI or EH level may come to understand via associative learning that shaking a finger results in a punishment consequence and therefore with training, may inhibit this behavior in the presence of this discriminative stimulus. However, the use of this gesture and understanding altered yet similar meaning gestures without training (raising a finger to gesture "wait" for example) would not occur. In another example, a common diagnostic sign for autism is the child not responding to his or her name, or inconsistently doing so. I would suggest that, like the child showing minimal referential eye-gaze or minimal enjoyment in social interaction, there may be a significant differentiation between no responding to name and some responding to name: the latter would indicate progression away from the PI level and would be a positive indicator. But the reason for non-response to name is the same; first, the child needs to be interested in what other people are saying and, at the object end of the continuum, they simply are not. Second, they need to know that one's name is a symbol for or representation of that self. At the object end of the continuum, neither of these concepts, symbolism or self, are present. Without these conceptual structures in place, why would a child at the object end of the continuum respond to a name? As with our previous example however, with time and training and consistent reinforcement, such a behavioral or rote response may become possible; but an understanding of a name as actually representing this imagined thing called "me" -- a self with likes, dislikes, emotions, and relationships in the world -- would likely remain out of reach. Similarly, the lack of pronouns use follows the same logic: if there were no imagination-based concept of "me" and secondary thinking "tracks" for symbolization, how would one be able to understand or use "I"?

Another common symptom of autism is echolalia, meaning repetition of the last statements made by others. Similar to this, autism is sometimes associated with "scripting," which is seemingly meaningless or nonsense repetition of books, commercials, or other statements that the child with autism has heard. Sometimes these are repeated over and over, usually in a manner unrelated to anything going on around them. Can we use our theory to explain this phenomenon? This is an interesting example because we can use the theoretical demarcations to note that if this behavior is present, we are likely dealing with a child who is at the EH or IH level of identification. This is because the symbol-based skill of language must be present, so we would expect this particular symptom to be associated with the corresponding, improved levels of functioning in other areas (some functional play, some increased awareness of and an interest in other people beyond the object level, and perhaps increased cognitive functioning over the more absolulte PI level person). But with only a partially functioning ability to think "about," that is, dual-processing representational abilities only primitively or incompletely formed, the internal voice that you and I commonly use and experience could only be poorly managed. Instead of seamless movement between the imagined internal voice and outside expression or management of co-occurring external stimuli, the internal voice may need to "be made" external. As a result, the songs, sounds, and statements that we can imagine on our second layer of processing tracks can't be consistently managed, and by necessity, internal becomes external. Given persistent focus on parts and a preference for constancy, the internal "clip" is expressed externally in a repeated and almost obsessional manner.

Another common symptom of autism that was mentioned earlier is behavior problems: tantrums, aggression, and self-injurious behavior (SIB). The object-based preference for constancy is likely central to much of this behavior, but we can use other parts of the theory to better understand why these types of behaviors make sense for the child with autism. Recall once again our robot example. If you preferred things in a certain way and these robot machines around you were somehow related to making things happen consistent with your preferences but now were not doing so, wouldn't you have a tantrum too? Now add to this equation an inability to understand the robot as a whole unit and an inability to communicate with the robot. There is really not much left to do but have a tantrum. You might even aggress toward this irritating and uncooperative machine and if that worked to correct the situation, associative learning would lead you to repeat the behavior. Similarly, SIB makes sense if you imagine parts of your body as disconnected things always nearby. For example, I chew on my pen-top when I work. This is a disconnected thing that is pretty continually nearby, but granted, it does not hurt as much as if I did the same thing to my finger. But remember, there is no unified, whole "me" in the child with severe autism, so hitting, biting, or picking at his or her body or otherwise doing those things that hurt would not really matter. The connection between body parts and "me" does not exist, any more than chewing my pen-top hurts me. As a side note, the absence of the symbol-based "me" suggests a more object-based identification, so consistent with this theory, SIB behaviors should be more prevalent at the PI or EH levels, as compared to IH or WH.

For reasons similar to those surrounding SIB, the common symptom of unusual sensory responsivity begins to make more and more sense. For the child with autism, incoming sensory stimulation would seemingly come from nowhere, which would be as unusual at it is unsettling. This is difficult for you or I to imagine because we objectively understand what our senses do, that they are an integrated part of what makes up the whole self, and what incoming stimulation of these senses mean. But imagine if that were not the case; imagine if every smell, sound, and touch had an undifferentiated, curious, unknowable, stimulatory effect that made no sense at all. It was only registered, much like sensing someone grab your leg, not being sure if it was your leg or your arm, and no one actually being there to do the grabbing. Beyond surprising, this would be confusing and again, possibly terrifying. As a general rule, one can imagine the likely preference for a quiet, consistent environment. Similar to this is the person with autism's tendency toward unregulated mood. Using our theory, I would suggest that mood would be regulated to the extent that the person inherited an evenness of mood; it is only with the ability to self-reflect, self-observe, and control our own reflective cognitive states that mood regulation can be voluntarily achieved. These types of abilities would only become available to the person at the IH and WH levels of identification, although there are exceptions based again on the associative learning model. Cautela and Groden (1978) for example have trained progressive relaxation, which is an example of regulation of one's internal mood state, using basic learning principles of repetition, modeling, and reinforcement.

So the continuum-based, dual concepts of inanimate object to whole human object and part-object to whole-object can not only lead one to hypothesize developmental effects, but they can help to explain some of the characteristics of autism that would otherwise appear divergent. At this point in our discussion, I would like to make very clear that I believe that the onus of placement or movement on this proposed continuum is predominantly in the hands of the infant, and results from the infant's inherited preferences and predispositions rather than being a voluntary choice made by the infant. That is not to say that environment does not play a role or that early, targeted treatment would not be effective but rather, unlike the original psychoanalytic attempt to explain autism, what the child brings to the equation may be most determining of the outcome. This perspective is not new to the psychoanalytic field, as reflected in a quotation from Blanck and Blanck (1986) in my 2011 article:

"Without this capacity on the part of the infant (merger with the parent), the mother's exertions are of little avail. Some infants, with unusual effort on the part of the mother, can be helped to extract somewhat, but principally it is the child who must play his or her part in using what the environment has to offer." (p. 15)

I would suggest that it is the interaction of the infant's biological predisposition towards object or human identification, impacted to a degree by the social environment, that determines the various trajectories we call autism spectrum disorders. To better understand the relationship between these factors, consider this graphic representation from our 2011 article (Woodard & Van Reet, 2011) (p. 223) (used with permission, Springer Publishing):

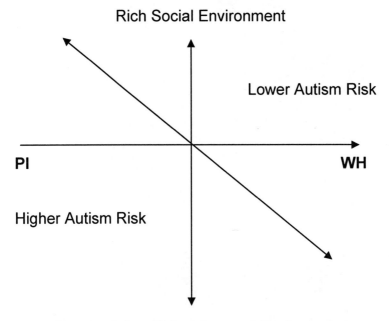

Rich Social Environment

Lower Autism Risk

PI   WH

Higher Autism Risk

Non-social or Object-focused Environment

Most but not all children typically identify early with human objects with ease and as a result, quickly achieve what we understand to be mature human thinking represented by the ability to think "about." This ultimately allows, at its most complex level, skills far beyond physical object knowledge/problem-solving or understanding the simple intent of others; it allows understanding even the most subtle social cues and facial expressions, complex person-based problem-solving, multi-faceted self-understanding and self-reflection, acute feelings of empathy and emotional alignment with others, and insight. I would suggest that a small, but apparently expanding group does not identify with human objects and to the extent that they don't, autism emerges.

Chapter 8: It Sounds Good, But Is There Any Supporting Research?

The title of this chapter poses a fair enough question, especially given the nature of many of the ideas that are central to understanding autism. We have discussed many abstract concepts out of necessity, in order to make sense of a disorder that to date has no reasonable theory as to where it comes from, how it develops, or why we see the variations that we see. But you may ask, "Is there any research that supports these ideas?" Because I have been thinking about this theory for some time, hardly a day goes by that I don't see a piece of research and say to myself (I can talk to myself because I am a WH identifier), "Of course that is what happened. It makes perfect sense if you think of autism as a result of object identification." I have tried to collect some examples here, although as stated earlier, I am often hampered by the participant group being simply diagnosed as "autistic." This is likely not a homogenous group as we have seen, although certain pieces of research identify "high functioning" participants which can be helpful. We have, in the last chapter, identified the more obvious, early, behavioral expectations that our theory would predict, and if you recall, early on we cited a number of research articles that identified the same behaviors: poor eye-gaze, poor response to play attempts and shared social enjoyment, poor joint attention/showing/pointing, using others as tools, and poor or no response to name. We have also discussed how this theory might help to explain both common and not-so-common symptoms, such as impaired language development, pronoun reversal, aggressive and self-injurious behavior, and even echolalia. But is there more? Below I have listed some additional behaviors, events, or outcomes that one would expect based on our theory, and what relevant research has revealed:

1) Based on this theory, we would expect that young infants with autism would be as interested or more interested in objects and object-based behavior as compared to people and people-based behavior.

And they are. It is already well-documented that children with autism do not attend to people, lack social reciprocity, and enjoy repetitive play with objects. These are defining symptoms of the disorder. Research (Hirstein, W., Iverson, P., & Ramachandran, V. S., 2001) has taken this one step further and measured the autonomic responses (electrodermal skin conductance) of children with autism when presented with a cup versus a person's face, as compared to normal control participants. These researchers found no difference in the autonomic responses of children with autism between the two presentations, although there was a difference for the control group. This suggests that for the children with autism, there is really no difference in terms of internal responsiveness between looking at an object and looking at a person. Interestingly, the subjects with autism were divided into non-verbal (27%), some verbal communication (49%), and normal linguistic ability (24%), which are groupings that could correspond somewhat to our PI, EH, and IH levels. Comparisons by these groupings were not noted in the research, which is unfortunate because our theory would predict increasing autonomic responsivity for the higher functioning group. However, there is this statement tucked in at the bottom of page 1885:

"Interestingly, we also noticed a trend towards above-normal SCRs to locking gaze in our higher functioning subjects, which we are currently testing experimentally."

Further, Klin and his colleagues (Klin et al., 2009) worked with two-year-olds with autism, and found that they failed to orient to point-light displays of biological motion. Instead of engaging in this essential behavior, the children with autism looked at non-social, physical contingencies (the same point-light displays inverted and played backwards). Typically developing children did the opposite and oriented to the biological motion; an essential behavior not only given the adaptive advantages of being likely to attend to other living things, but also the neural foundation for this behavior overlaps with brain regions involved in perceiving basic social information such as facial expression. Note that this behavior is typically present very early in a wide range of species, and present as early as the first few days of life for the human infant. That it is not present in young children with autism is significant, and suggests that non-social, object-based patterns were more interesting to this population than people.

Celani (2002) conducted a research project that shows the type of thing we are discussing in about the simplest terms possible. He had three participant groups: 12 with autism, 12 with Down Syndrome, and 12 typically developing children. Each participant in each group had four conditions with various types of preference choices to make: human beings and inanimate objects, animals or inanimate objects, pictures of a child handling an object and pictures of a child in contact with a human, and a control condition. Only the group of children with autism differed from the other two groups, and only in two conditions: the conditions with people in them. The children with autism consistently preferred the object choice over the people choice. And finally, Bodfish (2011) has suggested that autism is related to activation of the different brain circuitries for social versus non-social reward. For the person with autism, there is under-activation of the social area, and over-activation of the non-social area.

2) Based on this theory, we would expect that no single genetic marker would be evident, but rather that the more common genetic anomalies would map onto areas that could be hypothesized to be related to early, person-based identification.
And they are. We know from our earlier discussions that there is no single gene that has been found to be responsible for the emergence of autism. However, genetic anomalies common to some persons with autism have been found, and these anomalies are located where we expect them to be. One example of this is Ylisaukko-oja et al. (2006), who found that the best such genetic marker (D3S3691) was near a region of oxytocin-related regulation of attachment and associated social behaviors. And these types of findings have been found time and time again; Chakrabarti el al. (2009) located three autism-related genes in the oxytocin-vasopressin system, including OXTR, OXT, and AVPR1B. These genes are related to the emergence of empathy, prosocial measures, and trust. In a similar vein, Guastella et al. (2008) found that oxytocin levels played a role in gaze specifically toward the eye region of human faces.

This type of research supports the idea that in the search for a gene or set of genes for autism, the most likely culprit will probably be any gene that has the potential to affect the early human identification process: preference for human eye gaze, preference for object orientation, sensitivity to touch, sensitivity to human voices, preference for repeating movement or sound, etc. In a manner of speaking, I would suggest that there is no "thing" called autism at the beginning, but rather a set of predispositions that, under the right circumstances, affects the developmental course in a manner that results in a variety of traits and behaviors that we have chosen to call autism spectrum disorders.

3) Based on this theory, we would expect that treatment modalities that foster interpersonal engagement early would show an effect, mainly because the adult is inadvertently encouraging movement on our proposed continuum. This is complemented by basic behavioral techniques, the underlying cognitive foundations of which (associative learning and recognition memory) remain accessible to the person with autism.
In the early chapters of this book, I noted that effective, early interventions were those that employed established behavioral techniques within the framework of a pointed, person-based program. Popular versions of such models include Pivotal Response Training (PRT) and the Denver Model. PRT for example, employs ABA techniques and focuses on increasing a child's desire to learn skills related to imitation, language, and play. Similarly, the Denver model employs selected behavioral teaching techniques within the framework of an interpersonal relationship. But as we stated earlier, it is the one-on-

one engagement and human interaction that forms the centerpiece of many of these effective forms of treatment. No video, no self-management, no toys, no Skinnerian reinforcement machine, and no set of physical surroundings result in the same positive change. And the amount or duration of the therapist's presence seems to make the difference between effective and non-effective treatment. At least 15 to 25 hours of intensive treatment (accompanied by trained, parent engagement at other times) is an essential part of making these interventions work. In our next chapter, we will discuss how the present theory could possibly be used to maximize treatment efforts, and potentially further focus therapeutic efforts for even better outcomes.

4) Based on this theory, we would expect that there would be a lessening deficit in symbolic or pretend play as one moved up the proposed continuum.

And there is. While it is often difficult to identify where participants in certain studies might fall on our proposed continuum, research such as Wing et al. (1977) and Mundy et al. (1986) suggested that participants with autism had severely impaired pretend play abilities. These were marked by varying levels of impairment from an absence of pretend play to less spontaneous, complex, and varied (more repetitive) symbolic play as compared to typically developing children. In the Wing et al. (1977) research, for example, a total of 56 participants were diagnosed as having complete autistic syndrome, simple stereotypies and little or no social contact, no initiation of social contact, or repetitive speech, and only two of the 56 showed evidence of symbolic play. A full 32 of the 56 showed no play whatsoever, and the remaining 22 engaged in stereotypical play only. However, later researchers (Lewis & Boucher, 1995; Charman et al., 1997) found participants with autism who were able to engage in pretend play equal to that of matched control participants. While some of the participants needed to be cued and pressured into engaging in this behavior, more typical symbolic play was present in the group with autism. This research was particularly significant in the field of autism because it supposedly called into question the meta-representational explanation of the disorder. But how can two sets of research result in such different findings? The central difference was that the children with autism who were able to engage in pretend play were "high-functioning." Other research that supports the emergence of pretend play of children with autism also notes the role of the highly structured experimental environment, and the general lack of spontaneous play (McDonough et al., 1997).

5) Based on this theory, psychotropic medications designed to help organize thinking and decrease an obsessive need for constancy would be effective.
And they are. Anyone who works with families affected autism has likely been faced with the issue of medication usage. This is a particularly difficult area, because the parent has already had to struggle with being told that his or her child has a poorly understood disorder that is lifelong and often only moderately responsive to intensive, early treatment. Even with the best behavioral interventions, certain behaviors can persist that are dangerous to either the person with autism or those in his or her environment, and now the parent is being faced with having to discuss medications that are typically used for

persons with very severe mental disorders. I have had more than one parent say to me, "So now you are telling me that my child is crazy," or, "Are you going to make them into a zombie?" This process is, of course, difficult for the practitioner as well, but the positive effects that can be derived from responsible medication usage are significant. Behavioral psychologists seem to struggle particularly hard with this fact, and at least in my own experience, have often considered medication usage a type of behavioral "cop-out." For the behavioral psychologist, medications seem to be only attempts to "chemically restrain" or sedate, and while not typically stated overtly, there exists the view that medications are the crutch of the behaviorally uninformed and incompetent.

To a degree, there is a reason for this type of thinking. Aligned with Bettleheim's incorrect explanation of autism, the history of psychotropic medication usage is unfortunately marred by over-use of a relatively small group of potent and sedating drugs that were accompanied by serious side effects. Such a negative and evil-looking history has been further perpetuated by popular media, such as films ("One Flew Over the Cuckoo's Nest" and "Beauty and the Beast" are good examples). But the truth is that responsible medication use can do a lot of good (Myers, 2007), and when things go very badly, even the most behaviorally-oriented practitioner will call upon a psychiatric hospital. Today, 50 to 70% of children diagnosed with autism are on some type of psychotropic medication, and instead of sedation, reduction of behavioral challenges and improved accessibility to behavioral interventions are (or at least should be) the measures of success.

Over the past 30 years, the types of psychotropic medications available have expanded dramatically, and while research on their use with persons with autism is only now accumulating, the FDA has approved certain medications for the treatment of behavioral challenges and irritability associated with autism (Myers, 2007). Interestingly, these particular approved medications are technically "anti-psychotics," which is a term that can hit a parent particularly hard because of the layperson's knowledge of the word "psycho." But they are called this because they are effective with persons who primarily have disordered thinking, and associated mood and behavioral problems. That is to say, certain approved medications that show utility for persons with autism are those that help to organize the central thought processes, by bringing a calming order to chaotic and confusing cognitive processing. These medications are not designed primarily for mood, anxiety, attention disorders, or other mental disorders (although they can help with these issues in certain situations); they are designed for thinking organization and internal regulation. In our theory, the central effect of object identification versus human identification is on that very area, because object identification robs the person of the ability to think "about" to varying degrees. Without this ability, thinking can be severely impaired and disordered, and the world is likely experienced as a confusing and stressful place.

6) Based on this theory, infants who are on the developmental trajectory of autism should have unusual eye-gaze behaviors as early as the first birthday, and this should continue through the second year of life. Equal interest in various parts

of the face and other objects in the environment should predict autism.

 Research in this area of infant gaze is challenging, but we do have some evidence that eye-gaze is abnormal relatively early in life for the child with autism. Clifford and Dissanayake (2008) used retrospective parental interviews and home videos to explore early eye-gaze behavior and behaviors related to early expression of affect during the first two years of life. 36 children with autism were compared to typically developing controls. Anomalies in both eye-gaze and emotional expression were evident as early as 6 months, and became more severe as the child progressed towards his or her second birthday. In similar research, Jones, Carr, and Klin (2008) presented a group of two-year-old children with autism 10 videos of someone looking directly at a camera. The person on the video was engaging in typical game-like behaviors such as peek-a-boo. Eye tracking measures of the children with autism did not show the typical level of interest in the eyes, common to a typical comparison group and a comparison group with developmental delay but not autism. The group with autism's gaze toward the eyes of the person on the video was significantly less than the other two groups, and looking at the mouth (rather than the eyes) was increased. Further, the less the children with autism fixated on the eyes of the person in the video, the greater that child's level of social disability. In other words, the greater the non-realization of people as special objects with unique and preferred qualities, the greater the degree or severity of the autistic disorder.

7) Based on this theory, we would expect that children with autism would most likely have

physical awareness of their object-existence (especially above the PI level).

The crux of our theory is that infants with autism identify primarily at the object/part-object end of an inanimate- to human-object/ part- to whole-object continuum. We suggest that the degree of movement along this continuum defines how the person perceives the world and the self, primarily as a function of the ability to think "about" or imagine. At the most inanimate object/part-object end of the continuum, we would expect the ability to think "about" or imagine to be most impaired, and associated with a desire for physical object constancy, which would be supported by only recognition-based memory skills in contrast to recall-based skills. A desire for physical object constancy seems to come dangerously close to the concept of thinking "about" (because knowing that a thing is different suggests simultaneous knowledge of how it should be the same), and these concepts are closely related to research in autism on object permanence and visual self-recognition. As noted earlier, one would think that the skill of object permanence should only be present above the PI level, yet it also occurs prior to the behaviors representative of the 9-month revolution for typically developing children.

So object constancy, object permanence, and physical self-recognition could potentially go a number of ways in terms of our theory. Are these unique core elements of even the PI level of identification? Do they emerge separate from other thinking "about" abilities? Or are they thinking "about" abilities that correspond to our levels of identification? Another option to these being a function of a single thinking "about" skill would be that the ability to think "about" emerges in an increasingly complex progression. For example, the ability to think about an object continuing to exist where it was last seen or the same object being available, would seem most basic. Next, knowing that the object continued to exist but was moved to another location (demonstrated by a person continuing to search elsewhere for any given object), or all objects being in a certain order, would be more sophisticated. Understanding that the object changed its form somehow but was still the same object would be still more complex, and these types of rules could extend to people, such as wanting a person to physically always look the same or say the same thing.

It is currently unclear how our theory of identification would necessarily play out in this particular set of circumstances, given all of these possibilities, the comparatively early emergence of object permanence in typical development, and the unique role of objects in our theory. One likely possibility is that children on the developmental trajectory of autism may have difficulty in these areas at the most severe PI level, but beyond that level would have knowledge of the self as a physical object much as they recognize other physical objects. Research in the 1980's found that children with autism who were not severely cognitively impaired would remove a mark from their faces when they saw the mark on their face in a mirror image (Dawson & McKissick, 1985), but the experimental group of 15 children had intellectual functioning ranging from a severe deficit (IQ = 17) to nearly normal functioning (IQ = 89). This variation within an experimental group makes it difficult to draw conclusions from the results in relation to the present theory. Perhaps further research in this area would provide insights into this complex area.

8) Based on this theory, there should be some improvement in the comprehension or functioning of concepts that require a person to think "about," such as past and present, what "could" happen/fear, death, hypothetical problem-solving, or even lying, as one moved up the proposed continuum.

Again we are faced with the problem that most research does not divide participants into groups that would correspond with our continuum demarcations. However, there is research that begins to support these ideas. The area of thinking about past and present, for example, has been explored by Lind and Bowler (2010), but this is one of only a handful of research projects addressing these particular concepts. These researchers used high functioning participants with autism (which would correspond roughly to the IH level on our continuum), and found that participants with autism "recalled/imagined" significantly fewer events than typical control participants, and episodic future memory was also impaired as compared to controls. These findings are consistent with our current theory in that at the IH level, as a result of increasingly human object identification, these "high functioning" persons with autism can access impaired thinking "about" abilities. Interestingly, the participants with autism were more likely to take a third-person versus a first-person perspective in recalling events, which highlights the associated impaired concepts of self that would continue to plague the person at the IH level.

Similarly, high functioning persons with autism have shown abnormal (or impaired but not absent) abilities in acquiring a fear response (Gaigg & Bowler, 2007). In my own experience at the center where I work, we have a yearly Halloween party. One year I thought it would be fun for the children to have a hole in the wall, surrounded by a skull and a sign that read, "Put your hand in if you dare!" This turned out to be of virtually no interest to our students; each one stuck his or her hand in the hole without any concern at all, took the candy offered, and left. There was absolutely no concern over what might happen or what could happen. Further, preschool children with autism who had average intellectual functioning and vocabulary skills were able to provide alternatives to social problems (Bernard-Opitz, Sriram, & Nakhoda-Sapuan, 2001). However, the preschoolers produced significantly fewer alternatives as compared to control participants as we would expect. They were also able to improve upon this skill across probes which we would also expect given the thinking "about" capacities of this higher functioning group. And finally, while research is virtually non-existent on autism and the concept of death, the problem of persons with autism in understanding death and understandably responding in unusual ways, has been addressed (Forrester-Jones & Broadhurst, 2007). Taken as a whole (there is no known research on autism and the ability to tell a lie), these supposedly differing areas of research converge on one idea: emerging applied skills and concepts appear as one's thinking "about" capacities improve.

9) Others should be treated as mechanical tools and there should be more interest in parts of objects as compared to whole objects, again, to a lessening degree as one moved up the continuum.
Research specifically addressing the level of autism and others being treated as tools has not been

conducted to my knowledge. However, using other people's bodies to communicate (usually by placement of another person's hand on an object without a coordinated gaze) is a key diagnostic component of the Autism Diagnostic Observation Schedule (ADOS; Lord, Rutter, DiLavore, & Risi, 2002). The ADOS is the 'gold-standard' currently for the diagnosis of autism, and using another person's body as a tool is not only one of the coding items but it is one of the five scored coding items, meaning that it feeds directly into the cut-off score for the 'Communication Total' to diagnose autism. Clearly, perceiving others as objects to be manipulated rather than people is a central marker of the autism presentation.

Similarly, one of the diagnostic sections of the ADOS scoring rubric is "Unusually Repetitive Interests or Stereotyped Behaviors." This section includes any preoccupation with objects, repetitive use of toys, repetitive actions, and insistence on routines. But when we look closer, the example for pre-occupation with objects includes 'table legs' and 'wrist-watches;" not tables and arms of people with watches on them, but just the legs and the watch. To make this clearer, the scoring description for this section specifically states, "a clear interest in a part of an object." A number of studies (Liss et al., 2006; Mann & Walker, 2003) have indirectly addressed this area, mainly through researching what are known as "attentional abnormalities." In Liss et al. (2006) for example, 144 persons with autism were rated on a number of scales measuring attentional and sensory focus. What these researchers found through cluster analysis was that there was the expected over-focused pattern of attention in nearly half of the participants. This intensive over-selection of parts of objects was thus suggested to be a prime symptom of autism, and the authors review a range of possible neurological correlates.

10) Based on this theory, persons with a known, inherited object focus would have a greater likelihood of developing autism.

It is generally accepted that females are, as a group, superior to males in language abilities, perceptual speed, and verbal memory, and that females have faster language acquisition. Females have even been found to be more interested in facial than spatial or mechanical stimuli as early as birth (Knickmeyer & Baron-Cohen, 2006). Males, on the other hand, as a group, are superior in mental rotation skills, motor abilities, and spatial perception. While the literature on gender-based cognitive differences shows great variability across studies, these findings alone would lend themselves to a male predisposition toward objects. Baron-Cohen (2002) took this idea one step further when he suggested that autism was the result of an extreme male brain (EMB), or a hyper-male cognitive profile. In the EMB theory, female brains are characterized by a focus on "empathizing," and male brains are characterized by a focus on "systematizing." Empathizing leads one to better understand the emotions of others, while systematizing supports the ability to analyze the variables of a system which is related to skills such as visual-spatial reasoning. Again, with comparatively poorer people-based skills such as empathizing and language acquisition, and comparatively better object-based skills such as mental rotation and figure-disembedding (Falter, Plaisted, & Davis, 2008), if autism results from a tendency to identify with objects,

is it really surprising that males with autism out-
number females 4:1?

**11) Based on this theory, if there is any evidence
of parent commonalities, they should be in the
direction of inanimate object interest and poor
social skills.   However, given the theorized,
comparatively strong role of the infant in creating
autism, any parent commonalities should be weak
and non-universal.**
There is growing evidence that there is a broader
autism phenotype in families, which is a complex way
of saying that family members of children with autism
tend to have more subtle versions of the features of
autism.   A study by Piven et al. (1997) reviewed
research that showed parents of children with autism
tended to lack emotional responsiveness, show
impaired empathy, and display special interest
patterns and odd social communication. This was, of
course, not true of all parents of children with autism,
but with many.   Related research suggested that
fathers of children with Asperger's Syndrome tended
to show social deficits, and first-degree relatives had
significantly higher rates of communication and social
deficits, and repetitive behaviors. Piven's research
was consistent with past research, and found higher
rates of social deficits and stereotyped behaviors in
relatives of families with autism as compared to
families with a person with Down syndrome.   This
research supports the idea of poor social skills, but
what about object interest?   There is no known
research addressing this area specifically.

**12) Infants who experienced events that similarly
affected the identification process should have**

approximations of autism-related traits and behaviors.

And they do. If we consider the identification process, the infant with an autism trajectory theoretically brings a genetic predisposition for inanimate object focus, which is likely the function of genetic origins. Compared to this part of the autism equation, what the environment affects or induces is likely to be relatively small. That is not to say that we can't make a difference and should not try, but rather that given this situation, we need to maximize our environmental impact however possible; trying to affect the situation from the genetic side (by, for example, discouraging pregnancy for parents with the autism phenotype or one child with autism) would not be appropriate.

So, what environmental factors are involved in the typical identification process? We could hypothesize that emotion- and communication-laden interactions with the infant, eye-gaze, touch, reciprocal social interchanges, more person interactions than object interactions, and the like are probably crucial. If we wanted to inhibit this in some significant way, we could take eye-sight out of the mix; this would undoubtedly impair much of what is going on in the identification process. If we do that, is autism more likely to result? To explore this hypothesis, Brown, Hobson, Lee, and Stevenson (1997) studied children ages three to nine who had been totally or almost totally blind since birth, and rated them on a standardized autism rating scale. The results showed that 10 of the 24 children assessed met the diagnostic criteria for autism, although these 10 children were not quite the same as a child with autism. Specifically, of the 10 children for whom we assume the blindness "induced" a version of autism, only a small percentage had the same type of emotional and social impairment representative of a truly autistic presentation.

13) If a child develops autism as a result of identifying with objects instead of people, not only should they interact with others as if they were objects but their own behavior would be that of a conscious object.
Recall that in our theory, identification with other people allows us to think "about" in the most sophisticated manner possible, and to comprehend ourselves as people. It would follow then that if we identified instead with objects, we would see the world solely in object form, and conceive of ourselves solely as objects. While this is somewhat difficult to imagine, try to think of yourself as a thing only, with only biologically induced emotional states. If you were a conscious and mobile inanimate object as we are suggesting, how would you behave? We have already suggested that there would be little, if any fear of what might happen, so without supervision, the person with this thinking perspective would not likely avoid danger for very long. Further, not being able to understand the self as a connected whole makes self-injurious behaviors almost reasonable. But if we consider what we typically do to objects, a ball for example, we could hypothesize even further: we might slap it, bite it, throw it, spin it, squeeze it, shake it, roll it, or otherwise simply handle it. For the person reading this who works with people with autism, you are most likely saying to yourself, "Hmmm. Those are things I see in children with autism all the time." I can't tell you how many times I have seen a child with autism throw himself or her on the floor or against a wall completely without reason or warning, or how many times I have had a student ask me for

"squeezes." Children with autism commonly bite themselves, spin, roll, and love to wrap themselves in "body socks," "squeeze machines," and use weighted vests and blankets. We have all sorts of occupational-therapy-based, internal regulation theories trying to explain why this happens, but isn't it simpler to suppose that this person perceives himself or herself as an object and is simply acting accordingly?

Chapter 9: A Primer for Increasing the Prevalence of Autism within a Population and Future Directions

Once you have the idea of this theory, it's difficult not to consider what possible interventions might be, or to interpret new research, behavioral issues, or even current events without considering it. For example, I often wonder if we could re-initiate some version of the identification process to jump-start movement toward the whole-human end of the continuum. If so, does it have to happen at the infant/toddler stage, or could we make any progress in ameliorating primary symptoms by intervening with the older child or adolescent? Is it possible to basically change the infant's mind about humans versus objects, or if the child comes into the world preferring objects, is that the end of the line? Do we need to desensitize to humans, or simply reinforce early markers of human identification? Are we really doing the right thing by starting with the behaviors we do not see emerge, such as joint attention, or are these already symptoms of an earlier identification event? In the research realm, does this or that article show some intact, yet still impaired ability for the "high-functioning" to think "about"? What does the article mention about a preference for objects, or behavior that could be interpreted as that of a mobile object? How is the behavior representative of thinking "about" abilities? When staff talk with me about behavioral issues, does it help to understand why someone might be smiling at you while they spit at you if you consider the absence of "other" and the absence of "self"? How does the self-as-object re-frame the presenting behavioral challenge? Can we understand it differently or perhaps more as a behavior and less as a personal affront or attack?

Does this perspective change what we do... or could do?

Even with current events and cultural trends, I consider the positive effects of technology and how it might be used to pursue questions in this area, but also how the culture is evolving in terms of object focus. How is it different from say, 50 years ago? It is difficult to turn in any direction without finding some evidence of increased cultural object focusing. On a flight, for example, someone across the aisle was reading a newspaper article titled something like, "Up to 8 Hours: A Harmless Distraction?" The article was about how, on average, people now spend up to 8 hours each day engaged with a phone, computer, video-game or other "thing" at the expense of human interaction or just sitting and thinking or watching people. If we consider the possible effect of this on one's ability to do their part in the process of identification, is it really a harmless distraction? The article mainly discussed the potentially negative effect that this might be having on the cognitive development of the current and next generation, but I could not help but think about our theory and consider the implications of an entire culture being trained to engage with objects for increasing amounts of time on a continual basis. Based on this theory, one hypothetical way to increase the prevalence of autism would be to have culture-wide focusing away from people and towards objects, impairing the population's people-focusing and human interaction skills, and/or perhaps subsequently, impairing their ability to foster human identification in their children. Not only may the quality of interactions with children change, but the sheer time spent engaged in this essential process may be lessened. When the person reading the paper turned to me and said,

"Before you know it, we will all be computers!" I smiled back and nodded my head, and thought to myself that this was exactly the implication: we become that with which we identify. Or consider each time you turn on the TV and there is a commercial about how technological gadgets are all-consuming. It makes for a funny commercial to see people staring at their phones and walking out in front of moving cars as a result, but is this really something we should be finding amusing?

The most disturbing version of this that I encounter is when I am out to dinner or on a walk, and I see two people who should be looking at each other, not looking at each other but rather texting, checking messages, or something of this sort. Sometimes this is a couple for whom I wonder if this was all they had hoped their first date to be, but sometimes it is a parent and child. The parent is staring at their object of choice, while the child wanders about, looking for something with which to interact. Or, even worse, the child is looking at some electronic device. I wonder how much this happened during the first year of development, and what effect this type of culture-wide interaction (or lack thereof) has on this child learning to do the same. Will they find some other thing on which to focus? If he or she does, will this person as an adult become unconsciously attracted to someone who similarly prefers to look at objects instead of each other? What are the genetics of these two combined, object-focused people, and what might they produce? When they do produce someone, how likely are they to look at or interact with the child? Or will they be so busy checking their newest gadget that the child will really become more of an interruption? It is not news that emailing and texting has become nearly an addiction. Phyllis Hanlon (2010) reported that the

BBC had run a story about two adolescents undergoing treatment for cell phone addiction, and discussed whether or not such a classification as a disorder was truly warranted. But more importantly, she added that one-half of all US teens send more than 100 texts per day and 87% sleep with or near their phone. But haven't teens always spent a lot of time on the phone? The answer to this is likely to be a resounding 'yes,' but what is the effect of non-voice and non-person interaction at this rate, combined with all the other lost human interaction that at one time was in place in our culture? What does this type of experience mean for our ability to read the human cues of others? What does it do to our desire to engage the gaze of an infant? And is there any research in this area that we could look to?

Before we continue, let me again be perfectly clear: Autism has a strong genetic component, and there is certainly more to the development of autism than a cultural phenomenon where people happen to be looking more and more at objects. I am not suggesting that this phenomenon is the cause of autism, but I am suggesting that 1) it might be more effective and productive to shift our focus toward genes that may be related to the identification process (or objects versus human identification), and 2) we may be able to produce more effective treatments if we focus on any and every environmental factor that could affect movement toward the human end of the identification continuum we have hypothesized. Just like there are likely to be many genes related to identification in this manner, there are likely to be many environmental factors as well; what is most important is that we start looking for the genes and environmental factors with this theoretical framework (or a theoretical framework) in mind. Without a comprehensive theory, we are really just looking everywhere and anywhere without any hint of direction. With that having been said, we can return to our hypothetical discussion of technology-induced object focus as one possible contributing environmental factor, and then discuss implications and future research.

If we allow ourselves to view this as one contributing possibility, we have a singular example of how our theory directs us toward locating candidate reasons for the increase in autism. Again, this may or may not be correct, but at least we have a theory-based idea as to where to look. Consider the situation: Millions upon millions of people within a culture (and this applies to almost any developed culture, so it is difficult to compare one to another that is perhaps less object-focused and still has reliable rates of the prevalence of autism) are spending more and more time not engaged with people. Instead, for one reason or another, they are looking at things: computers, phones, or other gadgets, but not people. These gadgets are so consuming and reinforcing that the people in the culture really can't get enough of them. The more the people use them, the more entertaining, need-satisfying, and complex they become, to the point that some call them almost additive. Because the objects are communication-able and full of information, the people in the culture even put them in their homes, so in addition to carrying around mobile versions and using the same thing at work, these addictive objects are really accessible at all times and in all locations. As more and more time is spent on the objects, proportionately less time is spent interacting with actual people. Further, this electronic connectedness allows and even encourages the socially-challenged to enter the fray and become a part of a culture that previously was not particularly available. With the need for actual human interaction eliminated, anyone can become a player at least electronically, and what is created is a culture that is more comfortable with and interested in things than they are with people.

Add to this hypothetical phenomenon that half of the culture (the males, let's say) happens to be already genetically more adept at object-based interactions as compared to person-based, so they excel in areas such as spatial skills and object rotation. Further, the use of many of these objects actually improves these very same skills, and more of the group that was genetically geared toward them engages with the objects more than the other part of the larger cultural group (Terlecki & Newcombe, 2005). Not surprisingly, over time, a disorder marked by a preoccupation with objects and a lack of social skill becomes increasingly more and more prevalent within that culture. This disorder is of unknown origins and was at one time rarely identified or diagnosed. Also not surprisingly, the group that was noted to be genetically predisposed to objects is proportionately over-represented in the diagnostic category. Hypothetically, the culture would likely be naturally concerned with this course of events, so to compensate and correct what is happening, multiple attempts might made at rectifying the situation. Because the source of the problem is not clearly understood, researchers in the culture search everywhere for causes and try many different interventions. The only intervention that shows any effectiveness is typically developing adults spending many, many hours per week promoting person-to-person communication and engagement with the affected child early in development. Still, the cause of the problem evades researchers, and they ask, "What early event or process could be affected in such a way that a seemingly unrelated set of cognitive, social, communicative, and imagination-based skills are impaired to varying degrees? And, why is the nearly forced, intensive interaction with humans the only thing that helps?" I describe this as a hypothetical situation, but it begins to sound quite a bit real.

Future Directions

The hypothetical situation I have described above is one that we might currently be living. On the other hand, it may all be a coincidence, but doesn't such a large set of coincidences bear investigation? In my opinion, our hypothesized theory and its implications need to at least be explored. If we choose this avenue, there are certain areas that may be worth examining and certain things would likely be true:

1) <u>Symptom groupings would be present consistent with the four general levels of identification</u>: While the creation of the four levels of identification was somewhat arbitrary and created mainly for clarity, using an identification-based theory, we should see skills generally clustered together as described in this text. We all know that there is a continuum of autism symptoms, but certain levels of identification should enable distinctive levels of skill formation in a range of developmental domains. Using the identification theory and its corresponding hypothesized effect on the ability to imagine or think "about" should result in general sets of skills as noted in previous chapters.

2) <u>Object versus people focus in parents of children with autism/phenotype</u>: There is a phenotype that we

have described for parents of children with autism. This is not a "type" of person that is set in stone, but rather a general set of traits or characteristics that parents of children with autism tend to share. If our theory is correct, the phenotype would likely include traits such as a preference for objects, higher than average object-based skills, or relatively poorer human identification skills.

3) <u>Treatment would be effective to the extent that identification is shifted away from inanimate objects and towards human-based objects</u>: We already know that spending large amounts of time with typically developed adults who are specially trained to elicit social interactions and responses can have a positive and beneficial effect; we just are not sure why this is the case. It is logical given our theory that this would have an effect, but can we take practice and research even further and refine what happens during the therapeutic hour for the child with autism? If the theory is correct, certain other interventions used in conjunction with proven ABA principles should be effective in improving not only the severity of the symptoms, but the actual core areas of diagnostic impairment. These would be most evident on gold-standard tests that indicate the presence of autism early, such as the previously discussed ADOS.

Prior to starting any treatment, our theory would suggest that parent training and understanding of the ideas outlined in this book would be essential for progress to occur. Before someone can change their behavior even slightly, they need to know the nature of the desired change and why they are doing what they are doing. To further complicate matters, the necessary interactions may call upon the parent to be more intrusive, forceful, and socially-adept than perhaps they would prefer to be or perceive themselves as able to be. In addition to parent training, the child would need to be assessed to the extent possible on the more obvious possible sources of non-human preference or human aversion. Is it simply that the child likes objects better, or is there something actually aversive about the voice, touch, eyes, unpredictability, or movement of the human object? Autonomic measures during exposure to these various stimuli might prove helpful; both over-sensitive and under-sensitive responses would help to guide further treatment options. But using our more encompassing theoretical orientation and what we already know about autism and effective treatment, any intervention that falls under one of the following main categories might prove helpful in decreasing the core features of autism:

a) <u>Shifting interest and identification from objects to humans</u>: Interventions need to be developed that interest the infant in moving along this continuum, and becoming interested or even unified (to the degree possible) with humans instead of objects. The infant would need to be "met" where they are on this continuum, and then slowly shaped in the desired direction. This component would likely be embedded in a wide range of activities from the other categories listed, and would be represented in activities such as the presentation of videos that depict first objects, then objects with human emotions or traits, then humans with object traits. Expanding on this idea, any activity that suggests or promotes the changing intent and interest of humans (in contrast to the constancy of objects) would fall under this category.

b) Shifting conceptualization from part to whole/ 'putting together': Our theory suggests that not only does the infant with autism need to move from object to human identification, but he or she also needs to put together the parts of things and create whole understanding and conceptualizations. Interventions related to this idea would revolve around literally putting pieces together: beginning with objects, moving on to approximations of people (Mr. Potato-Head, animal toys, and then human dolls).

c) Fostering any "thinking about," representational or imaginative capacity that derives from (a) and (b), preferably from object to human: The categories above are suggested by our theory to be intricately entwined with this ability. Addressing all of these areas in conjunction with each other may prove to be most helpful. Interventions in this category would first, for example, pair object to object and then pair object to increasingly abstract conceptualizations of this 'real' object. In a related vein, promoting the infant to imagine the existence of items (and then people as in (a)) not seen would fall under this category. Interventions that prompt the infant to imagine the intent of another, see a matching substitute of the self, or engage with object to human puppets (for example) would fall under this category.

d) <u>Employing proven ABA techniques</u>: We already know that these work, so why not use them and integrate them into interventions derived from the categories listed above? The savvy parent, practitioner, or researcher will have already noted the presence of basic ABA principles noted in the above. For example, if we want a certain behavior to take place, it is unlikely that we will quickly get the 'terminal' behavior right away (especially with an infant). Instead, we will need to meet the infant where he or she is and shape the behavior by breaking the behavior down into steps (task analysis), and then reinforcing (or rewarding) successive approximations of that terminal behavior. Reinforcement of these approximations, appropriate and planned prompting techniques, and employing effective strategies such as discrete trial would all be examples of integrating known and effective principles of ABA.

Can someone really create interventions that are derived from these areas? Based on a feasibility study underway in 2011 and 2012, the answer to this question is "yes." They are listed and explained in Part III of this book. That does not mean however, that such interventions are effective; further research would be needed to determine if interventions such as those identified in Part III actually work. To empirically validate the efficacy of these interventions is an essential step that could take many years to complete, and they are offered here only as a possibility.

4) <u>Autism incidence would be reduced:</u> This should occur especially in populations without a culture-wide object focusing and reduced human interactions. In countries where this is present, the incidence would continue to increase. Stopping the upward trend of autism could only happen if human interactions once again took center-stage on a culture-wide basis, which is an unlikely set of events. This would mean that the culture would need to reduce or eliminate videogame/Iphone/texting usage, promote human interactions in place of objects in all environmental domains, train parents on the potential effects of non-human focusing, minimize the use of computers, promote face to face meetings and social connections, and even identify persons with the autism phenotype and inform them of a potentially increased risk of producing a child with a predisposition toward the autistic developmental trajectory.

In effect, we are suggesting a need to explore, re-ignite, or re-establish the human symbiotic state, and train the child to move towards (or at least tolerate) a human identification process. This will not likely be a pleasant process, but the payoff could be great.

There has, in the recent past, been a call for research that can clearly differentiate between interventions that affect disorder severity, and those interventions that are "deeply altering core mechanisms" (Bodfish, 2004). A quick review of the literature shows that the preponderance of treatment outcome indicators is more often adaptive behavior and IQ, rather than measures that focus on the three core symptom domains of autism. But building upon our growing ability to reduce certain behavioral challenges and improve for example, select communicative behaviors with technology, researchers are now being challenged to focus attention on truly desired outcomes, such as "children who spontaneously demonstrate more varied, sustained, and generative ways of interacting with their environments and with others" (p. 324). Bodfish notes that our ability to "promote characteristics like spontaneity, flexibility, and social understanding is likely to depend on our knowledge of the basic behavioral and neurocognitive processes that give rise to and support such personal characteristics" (p. 324). If we begin to think differently about the nature of these traits that you and I take for granted, real progress may become possible. If we explore the hypothesis that "spontaneous" behavior derives from apparently unique permutations of the thinking "about" capacity, "flexibility" requires a release from constancy and the ability to think "about" alternatives, and genuine "social understanding" evolves from successful early human identification, we may be able to move away from treating the symptoms of autism and open the door to affecting the core mechanisms that give rise to the developmental trajectory and resulting wide ranging symptoms known as autism.

Part 3: Implementing the Meta-play Method

Chapter 10: The Meta-Play Method and Other Models of Treatment

In the previous chapter, we identified various categories derived from DBT-A theory that would guide the development of intervention activities. In 2011 and 2012, a feasibility study was begun to determine if 1) actual interventions could be created based on these theory-derived categories, and 2) they could effectively be implemented by parents and with a young child with autism. We chose to work with two case studies, one of which is nearly complete at the writing of this book, and the second which we have recently begun. Note that this study was not designed to determine the efficacy of the identified interventions; we simply needed to determine if we could create interventions, and if our ideas could be implemented. Efficacy is a larger question, to be answered only through years of carefully controlled research. This means that the Meta-play Method has not been proven as yet to work or have any effect on autism. We are hopeful however, that in time research will support it.

We did not want to presume that the Meta-play Method was a stand-alone intervention, so we further researched other treatment models that have shown efficacy. One of those models discussed previously was Pivotal Response Treatment (or Therapy) (PRT) (Koegel & Koegel, 2006). To know how the Meta-play Method could interface with PRT, we set about identifying the main ideas put forth by this latter approach. PRT is based on a set of things we know about autism: the idea is that if one were able to "correct" this main (pivotal) set of concerns, other collateral improvements in functioning would emerge. Some of these main concerns included 1) a lack of motivation to engage in social encounters, 2) minimal social initiations by the child, 3) problems with self-regulation, 4) poor response to multiple cues, and 5) impaired empathy. As both a developmental approach and one that uses the principles and tools of applied behavior therapy, PRT puts forth an interactional style that is both related to and directed at these areas in an overlapping and integrated way. For example, it might be hypothesized that the lack of motivation is the result of children with autism not having learned the response-reinforcer contingency or relationship. Parents helping the child excessively create a state of learned helplessness, and hence the child then does not learn self-initiation.

The interventions that the Koegels suggest based on these ideas will be mentioned shortly, but note the basic theoretical difference between the core ideas of PRT and DBT-A. In DBT-A, I suggest that there is a single pivotal area that is foundational to all those put forth in PRT: the ability to "think about." I am suggesting that pivotal areas such as those noted above are not the core concern (although they are of concern), but rather problems that are derivative of early identification with objects that bars the development of sufficient "thinking-about" thinking. So for example, a lack of motivation to initiate and engage in a social-communicative encounter is not due to an impaired response-reinforcer contingency, but rather an impaired ability to imagine the thinking and emotion of the potential partner. Self-regulation is impaired because the infant did not imagine another person thinking of him or her, so the imagined sense of "self" you and I effortlessly maintain was never generated. Not responding to multiple cues is a function of not seeing the "whole" object or person, and hence one part or cue is focused on excessively.

Empathy is impaired because to have empathy, I need to imagine the other person's state of mind, and the main thrust of DBT-A is that imagination itself is impaired in the child with autism. And the imagination of human elements is the most complex and may happen much later, after object imagination is in place.

So the basic theoretical ideas of PRT are much different than those of DBT-A, although that does not mean that the interventions put forth in PRT might not show efficacy. On the contrary, PRT has shown good results. But what exactly are the main ideas in terms of PRT treatment? In PRT, the family is intensely involved, and treatment takes place in all the natural environments of the child. When interacting with the child, motivation is fostered by following the child's lead and interests, and providing choices and varied tasks. When the child does initiate or engage in interactive play with the adult, or even makes an approximation of such, the child is reinforced quickly with direct and natural reinforcers. Applied behavior analysis tools are apparent not only in the quick delivery of "reinforcers" and their use with "successive approximations," but also in, for example, the training of verbal behavior and initiations. To encourage skills such as these, parents and teachers are instructed to establish measureable goals based on the known and typical sequence of skills, create a clear opportunity for learning, model frequently, and reinforce immediately. The same type of approach is recommended for other desired behaviors, such as joint attention, pretend play, showing behavior, and alternation of gaze when making a request.

The PRT approach makes sense, employs known behavioral strategies that have been shown to be effective time and again, and focuses on core problem areas for the child with autism. I am a supporter of this approach, and I see it as completely consistent with the intervention approach that we created from DBT-A. However, I think it misses the central problem as I noted above, and is actually targeting behaviors and problems that are secondary symptoms. The other concern I have heard from parents about PRT (I have given many parents Koegel and LaZebnik's (2012) "Overcoming Autism," which adds more behavioral techniques such as "functional behavior analysis" and "replacement behaviors") is that the ideas and concepts are fine, but what do I _do_? By this, they mean that they don't actually know what activities to take part in, and they don't have guidance on what actual play to encourage. The Meta-play Method that we created is very different from PVT in this respect as well as theory, and lists a range of activities that infants can take part in throughout the day. The implementation of these activities can and should be done consistent with know PRT/behavioral strategies: model, reinforce approximations quickly, teach in all natural environments, create clear opportunities for learning, etc. The difference is, with the Meta-play Method, we will focus on a wide range of activities designed solely to 1) shift identification from objects to people, 2) move from part- to whole-object understanding, and 3) foster any and all imagination-based thinking.

To employ the Meta-Play Method, you need to know something about the behavioral approach and behavioral strategies and techniques. Explaining these is far beyond the scope of the present text, and the reader will need to access one of the many books or courses on behaviorism to gain a fuller understanding. A good one that I use and refer to often is Mayer, Sulzer-Azaroff, & Wallace's (2012, 2nd

Ed.) "Behavior Analysis for Lasting Change." It is also helpful to get hands-on training if possible, so the techniques can be practiced under supervision of a well-trained behaviorist. But briefly, here is a list of some of the basic concepts and techniques you will need:

1) Positive reinforcement and effective delivery of reinforcers
2) Shaping, chaining, and successive approximations
3) Discrete trial and errorless teaching components and strategies
4) Measuring operationalized behavior goals and tracking change
5) Ignoring and extinguishing non-desired behaviors
6) ABCs of behavior and contingent relations
7) Discriminative stimuli and stimulus control
8) Modeling
9) Generalization

Although certainly not an exhaustive list, these will go a long way toward helping parents, teachers, and others involved in the treatment of the child to implement activities effectively.

Chapter 11: Activities of the Meta-play Method

The actual activities of the Meta-play Method are, as noted previously, only recently derived from the ideas set forth in DBT-A. They await years of research to determine if they are effective or not. The reason I have written this book and outlined the activities now is that if I were a parent of a child with autism and someone had an untested idea that would not likely harm the child (and might actually help), I would want to know about it. At the very least, the activities of the Meta-play Method will give you some fun things to do with your child, and perhaps they will be shown to be effective. Beyond that, if the base theory is correct, perhaps others will expand on these ideas and come up with even better interventions than those outlined here. Currently, we have only begun a feasibility study with a small group of parents. We began by talking with prospective parents about our theory to get a sense of how easily the complex ideas could be grasped by people that typically did not engage in theoretical discussions. It turned out that our theory was not all that challenging for parents to understand, and the parents we involved comprehended the main ideas without difficulty. Parents were encouraged to offer any ideas they had for activities based on the theory, but this was a very different and challenging task that was mainly left to the researchers.

Once we knew that the parents understood the ideas and consented to participate in the research, we confirmed the autism diagnosis and severity with the ADOS. The ADOS was scored by a psychologist who was unfamiliar with the purpose of the study. We also collected information on the participant's cognitive functioning. With this information in hand, we began the task of creating a series of possible interventions. This took some time, but we were able to fashion a series of activities based on our theory and have added to these and revised them as the study progressed. Having nearly completed our first participant, we found that some of the interventions we came up with were simply of no interest to the infant, and others needed to be modified. As the study continued, we identified further interventions and were also able to place some of the activities on a continuum of complexity; our first participant was sometimes able to take part in a simpler approximation of our original idea, yet we wondered if the intervention in its original, more complex form might be appropriate for an older child, or one with a less severe presentation. So we kept most everything in our listing (each with a three-letter code), and delineated our categories for ourselves and parents as follows:

Meta-play definition: Items, interactions, and activities that foster movement on a developmental progression of the creation of meta-cognition, based on Object-to-Person Dynamic Behavior Theory (DBT-A). Five main concepts include:

1) **Any process of imagination from object existence to the more abstract human imagining (such as what others are thinking)**
2) **Any engagement that is out of the child's control or a product of (human) unpredictability vs. object predictability**
3) **Any activity that fosters movement on the object to human continuum**

4) **Any activity that fosters movement on the part to whole continuum**
5) **Any related or supportive interactions that capitalize on the use of effective behavioral principles, such as reinforcement or discrete trial learning**

Using this definition, we identified the more basic activities we created as level 1 and more advanced as level 2. These were revised and added to as our feasibility study progressed:

Level 1 Activities

1) **Pairing Reality with Representation (PRR):** (The idea here is to model for the child (and have the child practice and be reinforced for) engaging with dual versions of objects, starting with actual matching objects, moving on to increasingly symbolic matches, and then following the same process with humans.) Parents were instructed as follows:

   Pairing in natural contexts or matching in a planned procedure increasingly "symbolic" objects with real objects (the discrete trial picture version of this is more advanced (see Level 2 intervention) and should be attempted after actual objects are successfully used). For example, when you use a real cup or a phone, have the child initially use an identical version of what you are using. If he or she does this successfully, move on to you using a real cup or phone, and the child using a toy cup or phone.

Next, when you use a real cup or phone, have the child use a cylinder for the cup or a banana for the phone. Employ as many representations of reality as you can think of; one parent had a play "steering wheel" placed in the car, because the child was interesting in cars and driving. Try to capitalize on the interests of your child to motivate them to engage in this type of activity, and move only from real matches of objects you are using to symbolic as the child is able and willing.

In addition to objects, this concept can be implemented with representations of people. Create a picture or if possible, a doll representation of the child or family members. When you are doing something in the kitchen, for example, have the picture or doll do the same thing by acting it out in typical "doll play." Be sure that you have the child's attention and that he or she is at least attending to what you are doing. Move on to increasingly symbolic representations of people, such as dolls that are less similar to actual family members, "stick" people, or cartoons. These types of activities can be done in many contexts and locations, and should be varied as possible to maintain the child's attention.

2) **Fostering Imagined Existence (FIE):** (The idea here is to ignite imagination of objects, and then begin to move this ability to more complex or sophisticated thinking.) The parents were instructed as follows:

Training a behavior that fosters object permanence thinking, beginning with increasingly more shaded boxes under which we hide desired objects, and moving on to people. Reinforce any spontaneous searching for anything hidden, even when you start with the clear box. The goal is to have the child ultimately imagine that you could have put the hidden object or person anywhere, and for him or her to imagine possibilities of the object, and then the person's location.

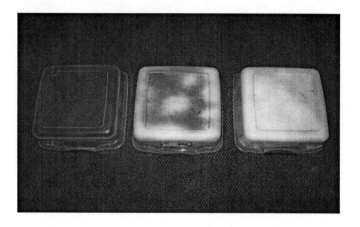

Sequence of this activity begins with the non-shaded box, then the partially shaded box, then the fully shaded box. Choose something that the child wants, and begin by placing it under the clear box. Be sure to get the child's attention and have him or her see you put it under the clear box. If they don't move the box to get the item, show him or her how to do this yourself. When the child can do the clear box, move on to the partly shaded box. Then move on to the completely shaded box. Shape approximations to the behavior you want, by assisting the child in getting the desired object as they approximate moving the box independently.

Next, move on to the child see the object be hidden somewhere in the room. In our research, we used a car that had human traits because the child was interested in cars. The toy car would talk, and then move on its own. We had the car "drive" under a blanket near the child, modeled getting the car ourselves, and then reinforced the successive approximations of the child performing this behavior. Once he or she does this, you can hide things throughout the day as the child shows a need or interest in objects.

After the child is successful with objects, move on to people. Let the child see you hide somewhere, and let him or her find you in the same spot repeatedly. Next, try hide and seek in various locations, reinforcing the child when he or she finds you. Finally, try getting the child to hide and you find the child. (The progression is from object to human, and from the child imagining objects to imagining your thinking.)

3) **Practice Unpredictable/Other-Controlled Play (PUP):** (The idea here is to have the child experience (and tolerate) objects and people acting unexpectedly and inconsistent with the child's thinking, to challenge the child to imagine where the ideas for this other-guided

experience was coming from.) Parents were instructed as follows:

Parent removes control and predictability in short to long periods with reinforcement, based on the child's positive and successful toleration or engagement. Begin with unpredictable toys such as non-directional balls or remote control cars, and capitalize on the child's interest in these. A ball that rolls in unpredictable directions may make the child wonder how this can happen.

Move on to swinging or "flying" the child where you are making the decisions on where you and the child are going. The goal is to make the experience fun, and have the child imagine that you are the one thinking about what is going to happen next.

4) **Staged Obstacle Situations (SOS):** (The idea here is to foster not only the child's understanding that other humans can do things (this can be done in a mechanical fashion), but also foster imagination of how problems can be solved.) The parents were instructed as follows:

Stage situations where only the parent can resolve/correct the obstacle and thus be the one that provides reinforcement. If possible, challenge the child to help you figure out a way to overcome the obstacle. For example, create a situation where a toy is out of reach because it is too high, and the child needs to come to you and ask for help. When he or she does come to you, move a small step stool close and see if the child can get you to use it. Try to reach for the object and move the step stool closer. By engaging in challenges such as these, the child will need to generate ideas on how to solve problems, which is a form of imagination.

5) **Restricted Parallel Animal/People/Puppet Play (RAP):** (The idea here is to almost force engagement with objects that are "becoming" more and more human, shifting the child's focus from objects to humans.) The parents were instructed as follows:

In a contained area, have the child only be able to play with or explore toys that are approximations of people or animals. This can include puppets or human-like objects and toys, such as Thomas the Train, puppet play, or objects with human trait play/animals with human traits.

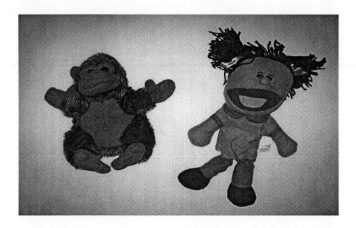

6) **Reinforced Putting People Together (PPT):** (The idea here is to focus the child's attention on the "wholeness" of objects and people, and away from parts, consistent with DBT-A.) The parents were instructed as follows:

Encourage and reinforce any play that involves assembly of human/animal/human-like toys, such as Mr. Potato Head, pop-up toys, or the bear or doll in pieces. Begin with whatever the child is interested in and will do; if he or she only wants to see the pop-up person come together, have them do that and reinforce it. If you can get the child to put one arm on the bear or doll, then reinforce that. Encourage successive approximations of putting the whole bear or doll together, and when the child does this, animate the bear or doll in an amusing way. In other words, make the toy come to life when it is whole.

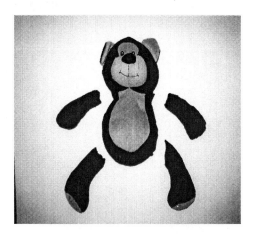

When the child clearly can take part in this behavior, have him or her put together a picture of the self.   Take a picture of the child or others in the family, laminate it, and then cut the arms, legs, and head off.   Using Velcro, have the child put them back together as he or she would a puzzle.   Challenge the child to "think about" this whole person; who is it? How can there be both me and a picture of me?

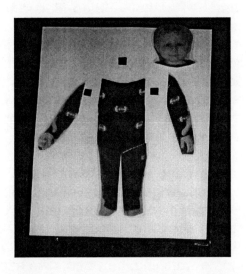

7) **Incidental Entertainment Training (IET):** (The idea here is to use a form of media that some children are interested in to further the ideas of DBT-A. Many cartoons and animated features have entertaining examples of objects becoming human, and we want to expose the child to this to ignite movement on the object to human continuum.)   The parents were instructed as follows:

Have the child watch videos where objects are people or have human traits, or those where objects are gaining approximations of human traits. Examples include the many household objects in "Beauty and the Beast" becoming human, the magic carpet in "Aladdin," the cars that have many human traits in "Cars," the robot becoming very human in "Wall-E," or shorter and less human shows such as Thomas the Train.

8) **Optimal Parallel Video-Modeling (OPV):** (The idea here is to 1) have the child see a representation of himself or herself, igniting the imagination versions of the self, and 2) effectively use video that was from the child's perspective to a) train desired behaviors and b) shift attention from objects to people.) The parents were instructed as follows:

Create a video where the mother is interacting with a matching substitute of the child modeled for developmentally-appropriate eye contact, gesture, social engagement and interactive play. Have the child watch the video and reinforce watching the video. An alternative to this intervention is creating a video that is from the child's perspective that demonstrates looking at people instead of looking at objects. Begin with a video of something the child enjoys interacting with and have a person call the child's name. Then shift the focus of the video from the object to the person and back to the object.

Another alternative to this intervention would be videos of examining the faces of the parents and other important people in the child's life. Begin with a detail of the face like the mouth or ear, and then shift around the face, slowly backing away until the whole face of the person is visible.

9) **Parallel Puppet Play (PPP):** (The idea here is to create in a format acceptable and interesting to the child, the idea that something else thinks. This thinking then needs to be imagined by the child. Using object puppets and then animal puppets and then people puppets, engage the puppet in joint attention activities or other interactive play with the child.) The parents were instructed as follows:

Start by using object or animal puppets that engage in what should appear to the child to be "joint attention" or interactive play. If the child will tolerate this, move on to human puppets that do the same thing. If the child hits or pushes the puppet away, pause with the puppet out of reach, and then restart the interaction. If the interactive play is too aversive, watching the puppet do things from a distance would be an alternative.

10) **What's in the Box? (WIB):** (The idea here is to prompt imagination of objects unseen on the object to human continuum.) The parents were instructed as follows:

Get a medium-sized, cardboard box, about 1.5 feet square. Cut a hole big enough on one side for the child's arm and big enough on the other side for you to place items in the box. Begin by placing items the child wants in the box and having him or her get the item through the hole for their arm. It is ok if the child looks in the hole initially.

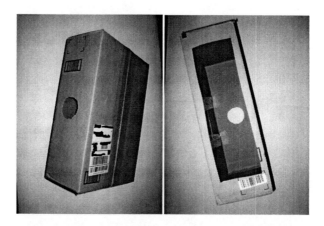

Next, have the child to select their item from a set of two items, the one he or she wants and a distracter item. Try to not let the child look in the hole. Then have the child choose his or her item from a choice of three. If this becomes interactive and game like, have the child move from choosing objects to choosing the more human object to get a reinforcer.

Level 2 Activities

1) **Pairing Reality with Representation (PRR) Discrete Trial:** (The idea here is to extend the PRR activity above to a more discrete-trial, two-dimensional format.) The parent was instructed as follows:

   Matching in a planned procedure increasingly "symbolic" objects with real objects by using the discrete trial cards (the discrete trial version of this is more advanced and should be attempted after actual objects are used). For example, have the child match first a picture of a phone to a phone (out of a group (array) of three items with two being distracters), and then a phone to a toy phone with the same number of distracters. The discrete trial cards should be attempted after actual object matching is mastered. Place the cards out and say "match." If the child chooses the correct card, reinforce him. If the child chooses the incorrect card, try the process again, but hand-over-hand assist the child in choosing the correct card. Run through 10 trials at a time, or as many as the child can tolerate up to 10.

Further information on employing a discrete-trial format is available in other sources, such as the Mayer, Sulzer-Azaroff, & Wallace text noted above.

2) **Acting on Other Intent (RAO):** (The idea here is to foster the child's awareness and understanding of the thinking of others.) The parent was instructed as follows:

Create a situation of staged obvious need. For example, place a ball beyond your reach and reach out for it. If necessary, say "I need help." Reinforce the child bringing you the ball. Try this again in this or similar situations, and try to reduce the amount of verbals. Your goal is to get the child to think what you are thinking, and act on it.

3) **(More advanced following successful PRR shift from 3 D objects to the discrete trial card matching format)** **Object-to-Person Discrete Trial Practice (ODT):** (The idea here is to use the discrete-trial format to reinforce attention and interest from object to person.) The parent was instructed as follows:

Use discrete trials where the target stimulus shifts from object-to-person. Examples include cards that you have that are on a continuum from a real car to a more and more human car, or a real cup, to a cup with eyes and nose, to a human-like cup, to a human in a cup. The child should be reinforced for selecting the **most human** option from a set of three, after you put out the correct card with two distracters and say "pick one."

These different interventions represented, in our opinion, the general categories generated from our theory (activities that fostered object to human identification, part- to whole-object understanding, and any imagination-based thinking). Each of these interventions could be implemented by the parents with ease, and the participants of the study would take an interest in them. Each participant's interest varied as might be expected of a 2-year-old, and interestingly, some activities were engaged in quickly and cooperatively, while others resulted in frustration and even some expression of anger and general distress. Parents recorded daily what activities they were able to implement.

These interventions were initially presented to the parents sequentially, partly because we were creating them as we were implementing them, and partly because we did not want to overwhelm the parent with too many activities. We found that we could present approximately 2-4 activities per week, so all of the interventions were in place by the end of two months. We found that we also needed to take some time to watch the parents implement the activities and correct any deviations from the original tasks. Early in our visits to the home, we completed a reinforcement assessment, and discussed with the parents this (which is a structured way to identify what motivates the infant and what he or she will "work" for) and some of the other main concepts of applied behavior analysis. For example, we could not discuss our interventions without explaining how reinforcement should be delivered, shaping desired behaviors, prompting, and concepts such as the functions of behaviors. Some might suggest that this type of ancillary training undoubtedly would confound evaluation of "purely" Meta-play interventions, but our purpose was not to evaluate the efficacy of these interventions. Further, the Meta-play Method was not designed to be used without other known strategies as noted in our previous chapter. On the contrary, the Meta-play Method makes full use of behavioral technology, and dovetails nicely with more widely accepted intervention models such as PRT.

How would you know if the Meta-play Method was doing anything? For our research, we repeated ADOS testing, used a global impressions scale monthly, and used a parent-interview every two weeks with the following format:

Parent Progress Interview

Child's Name: _____

Today's Date:_____

1) What kind of changes or new behaviors have you seen this week?

2) What new words have you heard?

3) Have you seen any imitation of your actions or those of others?

4) Have you seen any new gestures such as shrugging or waving at others?

5) Have you seen pointing or showing behavior?

6) Is your child turning around when you call his or her name?

7) Is your child smiling when you interact with him or her, or engaging more or less?

We were looking for any evidence that progress was being made on the core areas of impairment in infants with autism. Similar to PRT, we were (and are) hoping that by fostering attention away from inanimate objects to people, and from part- to whole-objects, we would be affecting _the_ underlying pivotal area of impairment in autism. By doing so, we would create the capacity for the child to "think about," and therefore the child would have the working cognitive capacity to imagine.

Closing Comments

I hope that this book has clearly communicated where DBT-A came from, what it is, and how the Meta-play Method activities derive from this theory. I do not want to create false hope in parents of children with autism, and would say once more that the ideas and interventions contained in this text have not been proven to be efficacious in the treatment of autism. Anyone who chooses to employ these methods does so at their own risk. But if they do help in some small way, or if this thinking is a catalyst for another researcher with a better idea that does help treat autism, then I think it has value. My only goal is to offer an idea that is complex, but sensible in hopes of improving the lives of persons affected by autism.

The author of this work makes no claim as to the efficacy or safety of the interventions contained herein.

References

American Psychiatric Association (2000). *Diagnostic and statistical manual of mental disorders (DSM-IV-TR)*. APA: Washington, DC.

Baillergeon, R., Needham, A., & DeVos, J. (1992). The development of young infants' intuitions about support. *Early Development and Parenting, 1,* 69-78.

Baron-Cohen, S. (1996). *Mindblindness: An essay on autism and theory of mind.* Cambridge, MA: MIT Press.

Baron-Cohen, S. (2002). The extreme male brain theory of autism. In H. Tagler-Flusberg (Ed.) , *Neurodevelopmental disorders* (pp. 401-430). MIT Press.

Baron-Cohen, S., Leslie, A. M., & Frith, U. (1985). Does the autistic child have a "theory of mind?" *Cognition, 21,* 37-46.

Bauman, M. L. & Kemper, T. L. (2003). The neuropathology of the autism spectrum disorders: What have we learned? *Novartis Foundation Symposium, 251,* 112-122.

Bernard-Opitz, V., Sriram, N., & Nakhoda-Sapuan, S. (2001). Enhancing social problem solving in children with autism and normal children through computer-assisted instruction. *Journal of Autism and Developmental Disorders, 31(4),* 377-398.

Blanck, R., & Blanck, G. (1986). *Beyond ego psychology.* New York: Columbia University Press.

Bodfish, J. W. (2004). Treating the core features of autism: Are we there yet? *Mental Retardation and Developmental Disabilities Research Reviews. 10,* 318-326.

Bodfish, J. W. (2011). Repetitive behavior in autism: Brain-behavior relationships. Association for Behavior Analysis International (ABAI) Conference Presentation, Washington, DC.

Brown, R., Hobson, R. P., Lee, A., & Stevenson, J. (1997). Are there "autistic-like" features in congenitally blind children? *Journal of Child Psychology and Psychiatry, 38,* 693-703.

Cautela, J., & Groden, J. (1978). *Relaxation: A comprehensive manual for adults, children and children with special needs.* Champaign: Research Press Company.

Celani, G. (2002). Human beings, animals and inanimate objects. *Autism, 6(1),* 93-102.

Chakrabarti, B., Dudbridge, F., Kent, K., Wheelright, S., Hill-Cawthorne, G., Allison, C., Banerjee-Basu, S., & Baron-Cohen, S. (2009). Genes related to sex steroids, neural growth, and social-emotional behavior are associated with autistic traits, empathy, and Asperger Syndrome. *Autism Research, 2,* 157-177.

Charman, T., & Baron-Cohen, S. (1997). Brief report: Prompted pretend play in autism. *Journal of Autism and Developmental Disorders, 27,* 321-328.

Clifford, S. M., & Dissanayake, C. (2008). The early development of joint attention in infants with autistic disorder using home video observations and parental interview. *Journal of Autism and Developmental Disorders, 38(5),* 791-805.

Courchesne, E., Alshoomoff, N. A., & Townsend, J. (1990). Recent advances in autism. *Current Opinion in Pediatrics, 2,* 685-693.

Dawson, G. (1991). A psychobiological perspective on the early socio-emotional development of children with autism. In D. Cicchetti and S. Toth (Eds.), *Rochester Symposium on Developmental Psychopathology: Volume 3* (pp. 207-234). Rochester, NY: University of Rochester.

Dawson, G., & McKissick, F. C. (1984). Self-recognition in autistic children. *Journal of Autism and Developmental Disorders, 14,* 383-394.

DeCasper, A.J., & Spence, M.J. (1986). Prenatal maternal speech influences newborns' perceptions of speech sounds. *Infant Behavior and Development, 9,* 133-150.

Fairbairn, W. R. D. (1941). A revised psychopathology of the psychoses and psychoneuroses. In *An object-relations theory of the personality* (pp. 28-58). New York: Basic Books.

Fairbairn, W. R. D. (1954). Object-relationships and dynamic structure. In *An object-relations theory of the personality* (pp. 137-151). New York: Basic Books.

Falter, C. M., Plaisted, K. C., & Davis, G. (2008). Visuo-spacial processing in autism – Testing the predictions of extreme male brain theory. *Journal of Autism and Developmental Disorders, 38,* 507-515.

Fonagy, P., Gergely, G., Jurist, E., & Target, M. (2002). *Affect regulation, mentalization, and development of the self.* New York: Other Press.

Fonagy, P., & Target, M. (2003). *Psychoanalytic theories.* Whurr Publishers: London.

Forrester-Jones, R., & Broadhurst, S. (2007). *Autism and loss.* Jessica Kingsley Publishers: England.

Frea, W. D. & McNerney, E.R. (2008). Early intensive applied behavior analysis intervention for autism. In J. K. Luiselli, D. C. Russo, W. P. Christian, & S. M. Wilczynski (Eds.), *Effective practices in autism.* Oxford University Press: New York.

Freud, S. (1917). Mourning and melancholia. In *The standard edition of the complete psychological works of Sigmund Freud, Vol. 14* (pp. 237-258). London: Hogarth Press.

Freud, S. (1932). New introductory lectures on psycho-analysis. In *The standard edition of the complete psychological works of Sigmund Freud, Vol. 22* (pp. 58-80). London: Hogarth Press.

Frith, U. (1989). *Autism: Explaining the enigma.* Cambridge, MA: Blackwell.

Gaigg, S. B./, & Bowler, D. M. (2007). Differential fear conditioning in Asperger's Syndrome: Implications for an amygdala theory of autism. *Neuropsychologia, 45(9)*, 2125-2134.

Greenberg, J. R., & Mitchell, S. A. (1983). *Object relations in psychoanalytic theory.* Cambridge, MA: Harvard University Press.

Hanlon, P. (2010). Excessive emailing /texting: The newest addiction? *New England Psychologist, 18(6)*, 1-12.

Happe, F. (1994). *Autism: An introduction to psychological theory.* Cambridge, MA: Harvard University Press.

Herbert, M. (2005). Autism: A brain disorder, or a disorder that affects the brain? *Clinical Neuropsychiatry, 2, 6*, 354-379.

Hirstein, W., Iverson, P., Ramachandran, V. S. (2001). Autonomic responses of autistic children to people and objects. *Proc. R. Soc. Lond. B, 268*, 1883-1888.

Hobson, P. (2002). *The cradle of thought.* New York: Oxford University Press.

Hobson, P. (2005). Autism and emotion. In F. R. Volkmar, R. Paul, A. Klin, & D. Cohen (Eds.), *Handbook of autism and pervasive developmental disorders, Vol. 1: Diagnosis, development, neurobiology, and behavior* (pp. 406-422). New Jersey: John Wiley & Sons.

Hobson, R. P., Lee, A., & Hobson, J. A. (2010). Personal pronouns and communicative engagement in autism. *Journal of Autism and Developmental Disorders, 40*, 653-664.

Horner, A. J. (1984). Object relations and the developing ego in therapy. New Jersey: Jason Aronson, Inc.

Jacobson, E. (1964). *The self and the object world.* New York: International Universities Press.

Jones, W., Carr, K., & Klin, A. (2008). Absence of preferential looking to the eyes of approaching adults predicts level of social disability in 2-year-old toddlers with autism spectrum disorders. *Archives of General Psychiatry, 65(8)*, 946-954.

Kanner, L. (1943). Autistic disturbances of affective contact. *Nervous Child, 2*, 217-250.

Kisilevsky, B. S., Hains, S. M. J., & Low, J. A. (1999). Differential maturation of fetal responses to vibroacoustic stimulation in a high risk population. *Developmental Science, 2(2)*, 234-245.

Klin, A., Lin, D. L., Gorrindo, P., Ramsay, G., & Jones, W. (2009). Two-year-olds with autism orient to nonsocial contingencies rather than biological motion. *Nature, 459* (7244), 257-261.

Knickmeyer, R. C., & Baron-Cohen, S. (2006). Topical review: Fetal testosterone and sex differences in typical social development and in autism. *Journal of Child Neurology, 21,* 825-845.

Koegel, R. L., & Koegel, L. K. (2006). Pivotal response treatments for autism. Baltimore: Paul H. Brooks Publishing.

Kogan, M. D., Blumberg, S. J., Schieve, L.A., Boyle, C.A., Perrin, J. M., Ghandour, R. M., Singh, G. K., Strickland, B. B., Trevathan, E., & Van Dyck, P. C. (2009). Prevalence of parent-reported diagnosis of autism spectrum disorder among children in the US, 2007. *Pediatrics, 124,* 1395-1403.

Leslie, A. (1987). Pretense and representation: The origins of "Theory of Mind." *Psychological Review, 94,* 412-426.

Lewis, V., & Boucher, J. (1988). Spontaneous, instructed and elicited play in relatively able autistic children. British Journal of Developmental Psychology, 6, 325–339.

Lewis, V., & Boucher, J. (1995). Generativity in the play of young people with autism. *Journal of Autism and Developmental Disorders, 25,* 105-122.

Lind, S. E., & Bowler, D. M. (2010). Episodic memory and episodic future thinking in adults with autism. *Journal of Abnormal Psychology, 119(4),* 896-905.

Liss, M., Saulier, C., Fein, D., & Kinsbourne, M. (2006). Sensory and attention abnormalities in autistic spectrum disorders. *Autism, 10(2),* 155-172.

Lopata, C., Thomeer, M. L., Volker, M. A., Toomey, J. A., Nida, R. E., Lee, G., Smerbeck, A. M., &

Rodgers, J. D. (2010). RCT of a manualized social treatment for high-functioning autism spectrum disorders. *Journal of Autism and Developmental Disorders, 40,* 1297-1310.

Lord, C., Rutter, M., DiLavore, P. C., & Risi, S. (2002**).** *Autism Diagnostic Observation Schedule (ADOS).* Western Psychological Services: Los Angeles, CA.

Lovaas, O. I. (1987). Behavioral treatment and normal educational and intellectual functioning in young autistic children. *Journal of Consulting and Clinical Psychology, 55,* 3-9.

Mahler, M., Pine, F., & Bergman, A. (1975). *The psychological birth of the human infant: Symbiosis and individuation.* New York: Basic Books.

Mahler, M. S. (1979a). *The selected papers of Margaret S. Mahler: Volume one.* New York: Jason Aronson.

Mahler, M. S. (1979a*).* *The selected papers of Margaret S. Mahler: Volume two.* New York: Jason Aronson.

Mann, T., & Walker, P. (2003). Autism and a deficit in broadening the spread of visual attention. *Journal of Child Psychology & Psychiatry & Allied Disciplines, 44,* 274-284.

McDonough, L., Stahmer, A., Schreibman, L., & Thompson, S. J. (1997). Deficits, delays, and distractions: An evaluation of symbolic play and memory in children with autism. *Development and Psychopathology, 9,* 17-41.

Mirium-Webster (2007). Mirium-Webster's medical dictionary. Mirium-Webster, Inc.

Mundy, P., Sigman, M., Ungerer, J., & Sherman, T. (1986). Defining the social deficits of autism: The contribution of non-verbal communication measures. *Journal of Child Psychology and Psychiatry, 27*, 657-669.

Myers, S. M. (2007). The status of pharmacotherapy for autism spectrum disorders. Expert Opinion Pharmacotherapy, 8(11): 1579-1603.

Perner, J. (1991). *Understanding the Representational Mind.* Cambridge, MA: The MIT Press.

Piaget, J. (1952). *The origins of intelligence in children.* New York: W. W. Norton & Co.

Piaget, J. (1962). *Play, dreams, and imitation in childhood.* New York: W. W. Norton and Co.

Repacholi, B. M., & Gopnik, A. (1997). Early reasoning about desires: Evidence from 14- and 18-month-olds. *Developmental Psychology, 33*(1), 12-21.

Rogers, S. J., Cook, I., & Meryl, A. (2005). Imitation and play in autism. In F. R. Volkmar, R. Paul, A. Klin, & D. Cohen (Eds.), *Handbook of autism and pervasive developmental disorders, Vol. 1: Diagnosis, development, neurobiology, and behavior* (pp. 382-405). New Jersey: John Wiley & Sons.

Rogers, S. J., & Vismara, L. A. (2008). Evidence-based comprehensive treatments for early autism. *Journal of Clinical and Adolescent Psychology, 37(1)*, 3-38.

Sandler, J. (1987). *Projection, identification, projective identification.* Madison, CT: International Universities Press.

St. Clair, M. (1996). Object relations and self psychology (2nd Ed.). California: Brooks/Cole Publishing Co.

Santangelo, S. L., & Tsatsanis, K. (2006). What is known about autism; Genes, brain, and behavior. *American Journal of Pharmacogenomics, 5*(2), 71-92.

Schafer, R. (1968). *Aspects of internalization.* New York: International Universities Press.

Scherf, K. S., Luna, B., Minshew, N., & Behrmann, M. (2010). Location, location, location: Alterations in the functional topography of face- but not object- or place- related cortex in adolescents with autism. *Frontiers in Human Neuroscience, 4,* (page count 16).

Stern, D. (1985). *The interpersonal world of the infant.* New York: Basic Books.

Szatmari, P., Jones, M. B., Zwaigenbaum, L., & MacLean, J. E. (1998). Genetics of autism: Overview and new directions. *Journal of Autism and Developmental Disorders, 28*, 351-368.

Terkecki, M. S., & Newcombe, N. S. (2005). How important is the digial divide? The relation of computer and videogame usage to gender differences in mental rotation ability. *Sex Roles, 53(5/6)*, 433-441.

Tomasello, M. (1999). *The cultural origins of human cognition.* Cambridge: Harvard University Press.

Tomasello, Kruger, & Ratner (1993). Cultural learning. *The Behavioral and Brain Sciences, 16*, 495-552.

Welch, K. C., Lahira, U., Warren, Z., & Sarkar, N. (2010). An approach to the design of socially acceptable robots for children with autism spectrum disorders. *International Journal of Social Robotics, 2(4),* 391-403.

Willatts, P. (1984). Stages in the development of intentional search by young infants. *Developmental* Wing, L., Gould, J., Yeates, S.,

& Brierley, L., (1977). Symbolic play in severely mentally retarded and in autistic children. *Journal of Child Psychology and Psychiatry, 18,* 167-178.

Psychology, 20(3), 389-396.

Wing, L., Gould, J., Yeates, S., & Brierley, L., (1977). Symbolic play in severely mentally retarded and in autistic children. *Journal of Child Psychology and Psychiatry, 18,* 167-178.

Woodward, A.L. (1998). Infants selectively encode the goal object of an actor's reach. *Cognition, 69,* 1–34.

Woodard, C. R., & Van Reet, J. (2011). Object identification and imagination: An alternative to the meta-representational explanation of autism. *Journal of Autism and Developmental Disorders, 41, 214-226.*

Ylisaukko-oja, T., Alarco'n, M., Cantor, R. M., Auranen, M., Vanhala, R., Kempas, E., von Wendt, L., Ja"rvela", I., Geschwind, D. H., & Peltonen, L. (2006). Search for autism loci by combined analysis of autism genetic resource exchange and Finnish families. *Annals of Neurology, 55*(1), 145-155.

Zwaigenbaum, L., Bryson, S., Rogers, T., Roberts, W., Brian, J., & Szatmari, P. (2005). Behavioral manifestations of autism in the first year of life. *International Journal of Developmental Neuroscience, 23,* 143-152.

CPSIA information can be obtained at www.ICGtesting.com
Printed in the USA
LVOW06s2115180914

404757LV00001B/192/P